NAMES
WE REMEMBER

Names We Remember

56 Eponymous Medical Biographies

C. ALLAN BIRCH

M.D., F.R.C.P.

including
ADDISON'S DISEASE
BABINSKI'S SIGN
BURKITT'S LYMPHOMA
CROHN'S DISEASE
DUPUYTREN'S CONTRACTURE
HASHIMOTO'S DISEASE
OSLER'S NODES
POTT'S FRACTURE
RAYNAUD'S PHENOMENON
ARGYLL ROBERTSON'S PUPIL
SIMMONDS'S DISEASE
STOKES-ADAMS'S ATTACKS
RYLE'S TUBE

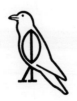

RAVENSWOOD PUBLICATIONS
Beckenham . Kent . England

Published by
RAVENSWOOD PUBLICATIONS LTD.
P.O., Box 24, 205 Croydon Road,
Beckenham, Kent, England

Copyright Ravenswood Publications
Published 1979

ISBN 0 901812 31 5

Printed in Great Britain by
Grammer & Co. Ltd., Vestry Road,
Sevenoaks, Kent, England.

Medical Biography Series

Volume 1
Life of Hamilton Bailey
by S. V. Humphries

Volume 2
Names We Remember
— 56 Eponymous medical biographies

by C. Allan Birch, M.D., F.R.C.P.

PREFACE

THIS book is a personal selection of short biographical sketches of some of the doctors whose names are often on our lips in current medical talk and practice. Many of the names are famous although my criterion for inclusion has not been fame but whether the name has become part of medical terminology.

Whether eponyms are desirable has long been debated. Anatomists have banned them and encourage, instead, descriptive, if dull, terms. Eponyms are useful when alternatives would be long and cumbersome. Examples are Menière's disease which does not commit one to any preconceived ideas of causation, and Parkinson's disease which is in common use instead of the descriptive term, *paralysis agitans.*

Other eponyms fixed in clinical practice are Horner's syndrome and the Argyll Robertson pupil. Of such names and the work that made them eponyms we can say with Byron

'But these are deeds which should not pass away
And names that must not wither'.

The past is neither dead nor useless and must not be allowed to be elbowed out by the present. It is hoped that these biographies will provide doctors and nurses with an historical background to their work. Lists of references are not given but a suggestion for further reading is made in each case. The short index will help in retracing items of interest.

Several collections of eponymous medical names have been made in the past. This one is modelled on that of my old teacher, the late Hamilton Bailey, who, with W. J. Bishop, wrote *Notable Names in Medicine and Surgery,* a third edition of which appeared in 1961. Two thirds of the names in that book were of surgeons but here the bias is reversed and only 18 of the 56 names are of surgeons. Bailey and Bishop contemplated a volume of

More Notable Names and I have used in a few of the present biographies some of the material they had collected and for which I am indebted to Mrs Veta Bailey. Twenty-two of the sketches were published in *The Practitioner* during 1973 and 1974 and I thank its editor, Dr Hugh L'Etang, for permission to reprint them.

I have received much help from many doctors, librarians and others and particularly from Mr Philip Wade, F.L.A., librarian of the Royal Society of Medicine, and his staff, and Mrs M. O'Brien, A.L.A., librarian at the Postgraduate Medical Centre, Hastings. Mr Bruce Eton, F.R.C.O.G., has translated German articles and advised me on the biographies of German doctors. My wife and daughter have read and improved many of the biographies.

C. ALLAN BIRCH
Salter's Corner
Hastings
1978

ACKNOWLEDGEMENTS

Acknowledgements and thanks for reproduction privileges are given to the following for the plates on the pages numbered.

The Wellcome Institute by courtesy of the Trustees 3, 9, 14, 17, 20, 23, 46, 49, 51, 57, 73, 76, 92, 105, 109.
The Royal Society of Medicine 11, 38, 67, 84, 151.
The Institute of Neurology 6, 156.
The Royal College of Physicians of London 141, 148.
L'Institut Pasteur, Paris 15, 16.
The Williams & Wilkins Company and Plastic and Reconstructive Surgery 53.
The Williams & Wilkins Company and Medical Classics 1.
Dr J. R. McMichael 32.
The Mayo Clinic 35.
Dr Stanley R. Wood and The Royal Society of Medicine 59.
The National Portrait Gallery 62.
Professor Hachinen Akita 65.
Archives of Surgery 70.
C. V. Mosby and The Journal of Pediatrics 78.
Georg Thiem Verlag, Stuttgart 81.
Professor George Grey Turner 75.
The Yale Journal of Biology and Medicine 96.
Dr H. H. Stothers and Annals of Otology (St. Louis) 99.
The Middlesex Hospital Medical School 102.
The House Committee of the London Hospital 112.
The Liverpool Medical Institution 116.
Annals of the Royal College of Surgeons of England 119.
Weber and The Lancet 122.
Dr J. S. Fairbairn and W. B. Saunders Co. 125.
Frau Eva Reiter 128.
Mrs Miriam Ryle 136.
The Practitioner 138.
Professor Dr Med. H. W. Buchholz 143.
Dr G. H. Whipple 153.
Charles C. Thomas Co. 130.

Each of the five living doctors named in the book (Burkitt 26, Conn 40, Crohn 43, McArdle 87, Sjögren 146) kindly provided his own photograph.

CONTENTS

xi

STOKES-ADAMS ATTACKS
Robert Adams 1791-1875

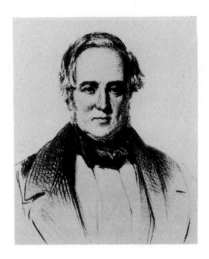

ADAMS's claim to eponymity is based solely on his brief mention in 1827 of one case of very slow pulse (see p. 151). Nothing is known of his early life except that he was born in Dublin in 1791 and that he entered the University at the age of 19. He graduated B.A. Dublin in 1814 when aged 23 and then toured the Continent to study under the best surgical teachers of the day. On his return he obtained the licence of the Royal College of Surgeons of Ireland in 1815 but he did not proceed to the degree of M.D. until 1842. He was articled to William Hartigan, a leading Dublin surgeon, after whose death he was apprenticed to George Stewart, surgeon-general to the Army in Ireland. When he applied for the post of surgeon to the Richmond Hospital it is recorded that his claims were so evenly balanced by those of another candidate, John McDonnell, that a second post was created by the resignation of Richard Carmichael who said the institution should not be deprived of the services of either of the candidates.

Adams founded the Peter Street School of Medicine and later the school of Richmond Hospital (later called the Carmichael School of Medicine). At the age of 70 he was appointed surgeon to Queen Victoria and regius professor of surgery. He was three times president of the Royal College of Surgeons of Ireland. He wrote a classic work on rheumatic gout, a condition from which he suffered himself.

Adams was a very popular man who enjoyed the society of his professional brethren. The Lancet referred to him as the last of the old guard of illustrious Irish surgeons of the 19th century. He died of heart disease on 13th January 1875 at the age of 84 and was buried in Mount Jerome cemetery, Dublin.

ADDISON'S DISEASE
Thomas Addison 1795-1860

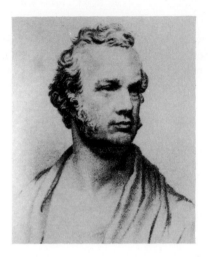

ADDISON's disease is chronic failure of the adrenal glands caused by atrophy of autoimmune origin though in the past many cases were due to tuberculosis of the adrenals. For the well-known clinical picture of low blood pressure, pigmentation and vomiting, Addison's name is always used. Its discovery was not a piece of clear-cut clinical observation but a somewhat confused description of what we now know as pernicious anaemia (for a time called Addisonian anaemia) and the disease of the adrenals.

On 15th March 1849 Addison read a paper to the South London Medical Society on "A remarkable form of anaemia". He did not mention pigmentation and vomiting but showed that in three fatal cases necropsy revealed disease of the adrenal capsules. Dr Pye Smith, of Guy's suggested that the anaemia should be called the "idiopathic anaemia of Addison". Addison did not distinguish clearly between the anaemia and disease of the adrenals and said himself that while studying the anaemia he had 'stumbled upon' another condition now known as Addison's disease. He called it "melasma suprarenale" and Samuel Wilks referred to it as "Morbus Addisonii". Addison's work was the first to show that the adrenal glands were necessary for life and it has been said that the whole of endocrinology dates from 15th March, 1849.

Addison's handsomely printed slim quarto, "On constitutional and local effects of disease of the suprarenal capsules", was published by Samuel Highley in 1855. Not much notice was taken of it in England but Trousseau popularised it on the Continent. Addison's reputation had already been established by his work on pneumonia. This showed that the exudate was in the alveoli and not, as was generally believed in the interstitial tissue of the lung. This study was a landmark in the history of acute lung disease between Laennec's discovery of the stethoscope and the beginnings of bacteriology. Pathology interested Addison more than clinical medicine and he was always happier in the post-mortem room than at the bedside.

Thomas Addison was born at Long Benton, near Newcastle-upon-Tyne, in 1795 where his father was a grocer and colliery manager. But his forebears came from Cumberland and he always regarded himself as a Cumberland man. Many Addisons had lived at Banks House, close to Lanercost Priory, and Thomas used to go to this house for holidays. The records of his early life are scanty but we do know that he went to the village school at Long Benton and later to the grammar school at Newcastle-upon-Tyne. He learned Latin so well that he spoke it fluently and used it to make his lecture notes. His father wished him to take up law but Thomas preferred medicine. So he refused to work in a lawyer's office and went straight to Edinburgh University where he graduated M.D. in 1815. He then came to London where, although qualified, he entered Guy's Hospital as an ordinary student. He became L.R.C.P. in 1819 and a Fellow, unusually late, in 1838. He never held office at the College. An early appointment was that of physician to the General Dispensary and in 1824 he became assistant physician to Guy's Hospital, attaining the rank of full physician in 1837.

Addison was a brilliant and popular lecturer and his students

4

worshipped him. Although sometimes haughty and unapproachable this was just a cloak for his nervousness. His story has a note of sadness in it. He did not build up a large practice and was almost unknown to the public. He was a sensitive and unhappy man, full of doubt and self-criticism. The story is told that on one occasion, after seeing a patient outside London, he posted back many miles to satisfy himself about some doubt which had arisen in his mind. He suffered much from insomnia. None of the usual honours such as Fellowship of the Royal Society, honorary degrees and Court appointments came his way and his fame is mainly posthumous. He had always had "fits of awful despondency" and towards the end of his life he suffered from gallstones and jaundice. He resigned his post at Guy's in March 1860, despite pleas from his students to stay on, knowing that he was probably faced with serious mental illness. He had married in 1847, when aged 52, Elizabeth Hauxwell, a widow with two children, but he had none of his own. On his retirement they went to live at 15 Wellington Villas, Brighton. There he had two constant attendants but managed to elude them and jumped into the area nine feet below. He died about 12 hours later, having fractured his skull. The coroner's verdict was "accidental death" but there seems no doubt that the basic cause was depression. He was buried at Lanercost Priory. An obituary notice appeared in only one paper, The Medical Times and Gazette. Yet his name is now well known for the disease named after him.

A stained glass window in the organ chamber of Long Benton Church, though undedicated, was installed in his memory. A memorial plaque was placed in the church and there are busts at Guy's Hospital and in the Royal College of Physicians of London.

ADIE'S PUPIL
William John Adie 1886-1935

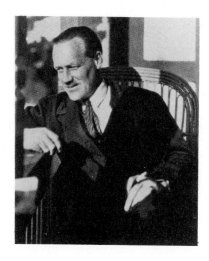

THE pupil which reacts to accommodation but not to light had been described by Argyll Robertson in 1869 (see p. 130) and was always attributed to syphilis of the central nervous system. Adie, a careful clinical observer, interested in the ambiguity of certain physical signs, recognised a pupil which resembled that described by Argyll Robertson but differed from it in important respects. It was unilateral and only reacted slowly to accommodation. Although it appeared not to react to light it did so after the patient had been in the dark for a long time. It responded normally by dilatation with mydriatics. It was called the "tonic pupil" and when it was associated with congenital absence of tendon reflexes the picture presented was called pseudo-tabes. Adie's account of the condition was published in the British Medical Journal 1931 2 136 and also in another paper in Brain (1932 55 98). Gordon Holmes was very interested in the condition, too, and published a paper on Partial Iridoplegia (Transactions of the

Ophthalmological Society of the United Kingdom 1931 51 209).
He said the tonic pupil showed a "myotonia-like reaction" and
that there were virtually no other symptoms and signs. The
condition is therefore sometimes called the Holmes-Adie pupil.
Adie wrote on many neurological subjects — pituitary tumours,
disseminated sclerosis and idiopathic narcolepsy, a condition
sometimes referred to eponymously by the French as "maladie
d'Adie".

William John Adie was born at Geelong, Australia, on 31st
October 1886, the eldest son of David Adie, and was educated at
Flinders School there. He graduated at Edinburgh in 1911. His
medical career was interrupted by World War I. In 1914 he went to
France as medical officer to the Northamptonshire Regiment and
was one of its few survivors in the retreat from Mons. Always
interested in neurology, he soon became neurological specialist to
the 7th General Hospital. When the war ended Adie became
medical registrar at Charing Cross Hospital and went on to obtain
higher qualifications: M.R.C.P. in 1919 and M.D. with gold
medal in 1920. He was elected F.R.C.P. in 1925. He served on the
staff of several London hospitals — the Royal Northern, the
National Hospital for Nervous Diseases (see footnote p. 156), the
Royal London Ophthalmic Hospital and Mount Vernon
Hospital.

Adie was endowed with a sympathetic outlook on life and had
all the qualities of an ideal consultant. He possessed the art of
summarising complex problems with clarity and elegance.
Perhaps his most endearing characteristic was his
approachability. He was entirely free from affectation and never
assumed the distant manner that sometimes afflicted those who
were too conscious of their status as physicians to the great
teaching hospitals. Perhaps his close personal contact with his
students had its origin in his colonial upbringing. Students
benefited greatly from it, for he was just as ready to discuss a
medical problem with them as with his senior colleagues.
Without a rival as a clinical teacher, he was a Sherlock Holmes at
the bedside where he used to the full his deductions from the
clinical signs he elicited. He was well aware of this and would
recount with pardonable pride the fact that he had "spotted" a
man's occupation as a wine waiter by the way he walked into the

room. Adie made diagnosis look easy. He did not fly to ancillary help or take refuge behind laboratory reports, using these rather to check and confirm his clinically-made decisions. Another asset was his mastery of foreign languages. He made a point of keeping up-to-date with German periodicals and said this gave him an advantage over his colleagues.

Adie married Lorraine Bonar, of Edinburgh, in 1916, and they had a son and a daughter. It is sad to record that he died of coronary thrombosis on 17th March, 1935 at the early age of 48, having been ill for three years.

BABINSKI'S SIGN
Joseph Francois Felix Babinski 1857-1932

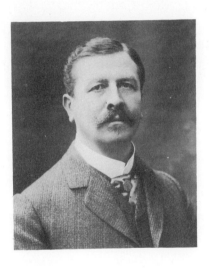

EVERY house physician in his routine examination of a patient looks for Babinski's sign as he strokes the soles of the feet with the end of his patellar hammer or his door key. He may record the result as "plantars extensor" but he knows that the sign he elicits is named after Babinski. This famous sign, or "cutaneous plantar reflex", was described in a communication of only 28 lines to a meeting of the Société de Biologie in 1896. (Comptes rendus hebdomadaires des séances de la Société de Biologie, Paris, 1896 3 207). It simply stated that in certain cases of organic disease of the central nervous system stimulation of the soles causes extension of the great toe instead of the normal flexion. The associated fanning of the toes (signe de l'éventail) was added in 1903. Dorsiflexion of the great toe had been reported three years earlier by E. Remak but it was Babinski who realised its diagnostic significance.

Babinski's parents were political refugees from Poland and he was born in Paris where he graduated in medicine in 1884. He

9

worked under Charcot at the Salpêtrière and from 1890 to 1927 was head of the neurological clinic at the Hopital de la Pitié. He was very different from Charcot, lacking his master's clinical flair, and, as he did not succeed in the competitive examination for the title, professeur agrégé, he did not become his successor. So he did not have to hold systematic teaching sessions as Charcot had done, but he followed his master in holding clinical lecture demonstrations. His method was that of meticulous scrutiny and consideration of the clinical problem with little use of ancillary aids, deploring snap diagnosis. Our present-day routine neurological examination is largely that of Babinski. He wrote articles regularly and his bibliography contains 288 items. Like Charcot, Babinski became interested in hysteria which, he said, was due to suggestion. He was one of the first to note that many of the symptoms of hysterical patients at the Salpêtrière vanished when Charcot died.

Babinski was a good histologist as well as a clinician. He foresaw the advent of neurosurgery and said he regarded his best contribution to neurology to be not his famous sign but that he had shown the way to the early French neurosurgeons, de Martel and Clovis Vincent. He himself assisted his colleague, Lecène, to remove the first spinal cord tumour to be operated on in France.

Over six feet tall and a man of few words, Babinski had a formidable presence. He frequently attended the opera and ballet. He had a passion for good food and there is a story that he once interrupted his ward round and dashed home when the ward sister gave him a message that the soufflé was nearing perfection. Babinski died in Paris at the age of 75, his later years having been marred by Parkinson's disease.

BELL'S PALSY
Sir Charles Bell 1774-1842

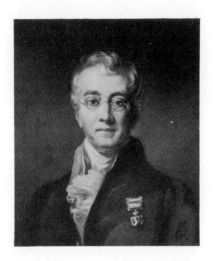

In the familiar Bell's palsy the function of the seventh cranial or facial nerve is interrupted so that the face becomes asymetrical. The eye cannot be closed and, as the corner of the mouth is paralysed, there is difficulty in articulation and in drinking. Interference with the nervous pathway above the facial nerve or upper motor neurone facial paralysis only affects the lower face. This kind of facial paralysis is not included in the term Bell's palsy.

The career of the man who described facial paralysis is an example of how brilliance overcame many obstacles and brought fame in the end. Bell's father, The Rev. William Bell, of Doune, Perthshire, died when Charles was only five years old. This early handicap was overcome by Charles's mother who taught him till he was 14 when he attended the Edinburgh High School. He described his two years there as "Torture and humiliation" and, opposite a statement in Pettigrew's Medical Portrait Gallery that he was educated there, he wrote: "Nonsense, I received no education but from my mother, neither reading, writing, cyphering nor anything else". She was a talented artist. That she passed on her artistic ability to her son is shown by the fact that Charles, who qualified in 1799, published, while still a student, a System of Dissections, illustrated by his own drawings. His brother, eleven years his senior, was a successful Edinburgh surgeon, but jealousy of the pair involved them in a feud with the Medical Faculty of Edinburgh. This resulted in their being denied further positions in the University and forced Charles to go to London. There he soon published his *magnum opus*, "On the Anatomy and Philosophy of Expression" (Longmans 1806), a book for the instruction of artists. He presented a copy to Queen Charlotte, wife of George III. This successful venture brought him immediate recognition in art circles and in the social life of London. It secured for him the anatomical chair at the Royal Academy. He taught anatomy at the Great Windmill Street School (now the site of the Lyric Theatre), which William Hunter had started, and by 1812 was its proprietor.

Bell studied the hitherto neglected subject of the anatomy of nerves and demonstrated that motor nerves ran in the anterior roots of the spinal cord. The pathway of sensory fibres in the posterior roots had already been shown by Magendie. Nevertheless, the routes of sensory and motor fibres are still referred to as being governed by Bell's law. He also showed that the nerves of special senses could be traced from specific areas in the brain to the end organs and that the fifth cranial nerve was motor to mastication and sensory to the face, whereas the seventh nerve controlled the muscles of expression. These were all fundamental discoveries which we now take for granted. Seventh nerve paralysis of the lower motor neurone type is generally called Bell's palsy to this day. Bell's paper, "On the Nerves; giving an account of some experiments on their structure and functions which lead to a new arrangement of the system", was read on 21st July 1821 and published in the Philosophical Transactions of the Royal Society, London 1821 111 398. Bell's "Nervous system of the Human Body", the first textbook of modern neurology, appeared in 1830.

In 1813 Bell became a Member of the Royal College of Surgeons (then of London) and in 1825 was professor of anatomy and surgery in the College. At the height of his career he was instrumental in founding the Middlesex Hospital and Medical School. After the Battle of Waterloo in 1815 he went to Brussels to take charge of a hospital where he operated on large numbers of wounded until his clothes were "stiff with blood". Many honours came to Bell, including a knighthood in 1831. Towards the end of his life he decided to leave London, considering that "London was a good place to live in but not to die in", and in 1835 he took up the post of professor of surgery in his native city. But his health began to fail and he had frequent attacks of angina. He came south with his wife in 1842 to stay with a close friend, Mrs Holland, at Hallow, Worcestershire, but died two days after arrival. He was buried in the churchyard there.

Bell was a genial man with a twinkle in his eye and quite unaffected. He lacked business acumen and perhaps that is why, despite his abilities, he never achieved affluence. His widow, formerly Marion Shaw, of Ayr, was so poor that a Civil List pension of £100 was awarded to her. He is said to have disposed of his very valuable museum of anatomical and surgical specimens to the Royal College of Surgeons of Edinburgh for the small sum of £3,000. He was referred to as "good kind-hearted, happy Charlie Bell", and one of his friends said of him: "If ever I knew a genuinely and practically happy man it was Sir Charles Bell".

BOWMAN'S MEMBRANE
BOWMAN'S CAPSULE
Sir William Bowman Bart 1816-1892

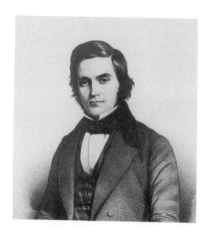

THIS distinguished surgeon's name is commemorated in at least two unrelated branches of medicine, namely ophthalmology and renal physiology. But his discoveries in these spheres remind us of only a few of the great contributions he made to medicine. They illustrate the high qualities with which he was endowed.

He was born at Nantwich, Cheshire, on 20th July 1816. His father, a banker, was also a botanist and geologist and his mother a fine draughtswoman and painter. William, the third of three sons, was educated at Hazelwood School, Birmingham, famous then for the fact that it did not use corporal punishment and was successfully governed by the boys themselves. The study of natural science was encouraged. He became head boy and, while experimenting with gunpowder, he injured his hand. He was so impressed by the care he received from a surgeon, Mr Joseph Hodgson (who became P.R.C.S. in 1864), and so interested in the wound itself that he decided to become a doctor. He was apprenticed for five years at a fee of 100 guineas to Mr Hodgson, who gave him a microscope in recognition of his industry. In Bowman's time a period at one of the London hospitals was necessary to qualify and so he worked at King's College Hospital. He became M.R.C.S. in 1839 and a Fellow in 1844. He was soon assistant surgeon at King's College Hospital and became full surgeon by 1856. In 1846 he had been appointed surgeon to the Royal London Ophthalmic Hospital in Moorfields. He became more and more involved in eye work in which he was a pioneer, being the first, for example, to use the ophthalmoscope invented by Helmholtz in 1851. Although he protested that he was a general surgeon, there was not enough work in this sphere to share in competition with his fellows and he gradually relinquished all surgery outside the field of ophthalmology.

In Bowman's time microscopes were primitive and sections were cut by hand, as microtomes were unknown. Bowman's skill won him a reputation as a first-class microscopist before he was 26 and earned him the title of "Father of General Anatomy" (later called histology). On 18th June 1840 he read a paper to the Royal Society, "On the structure and movements of voluntary muscle", and this secured his election to be F.R.S. at the age of 25. A paper, "On the structure and use of the Malpighian bodies of the kidneys with observations on the circulation through that gland", on 17th February 1842, gained him the Royal Medal. Bowman was the first to show that each renal tubule had a dilated blind end (Bowman's capsule) pushed in by a tuft of "capillaries" (the glomerulus). Although the Malpighian body was known, it was left to Bowman to show its structure and all studies of renal function can be said to have originated in his work.

Most of Bowman''s life was spent in the practice of ophthalmology to which the dexterity of his thin fingers suited him. His work in this field is commemorated in Bowman's membrane, the homogeneous basement membrance between the corneal epithelium and the main mass of the cornea. He made many other discoveries — the ciliary muscle and the glands of the nasal mucuous membrance — and invented many instruments such as Bowman's probe.

Now that the knowledge resulting from much of Bowman's

work is commonplace it is hard to appreciate the true greatness of the man and how much he added to our knowledge of physiological histology and ophthalmology. His work as a physiologist is commemorated in Birmingham University in the title, Bowman Professor of Physiology. A disposition for earnest study and high mental and moral culture prevailed in his home as a young man and he had the natural ability to concentrate all his thoughts on the subject he was investigating. He took great pride in his chosen profession. In later life his air of dignity and the calmness of his movement and speech suggested power in reserve. He was an abstemious man, eating little, drinking less and not smoking at all. He was an early riser and it is recorded that it was his habit to do some gardening work before going to his rooms in London. He was of slender build and not robust, though rarely ill. His tranquil home at Hampstead was full of works of art and he preferred being there to spending late nights at social occasions. He was deeply religious and could recite the psalms from memory and nearly all the writings of St John. He was wonderfully kind to all his patients and treated gratis many in poor circumstances. He had all the Victorian virtues. As a teacher he was painstaking, and lectured slowly to allow his students to take notes. Many honours came to him, including a baronetcy in 1884. Bowman married in 1842 his cousin, Harriet Paget, the fifth daughter of a surgeon of Leicester, and they had seven children. In later life he lived at Joldwynds, near Dorking, where he died on 20th March 1892, aged 76, a week after his complete retirement from practice. He was buried at Holmbury St Mary.

BROCA'S AREA
Pierre-Paul Broca 1824-1880

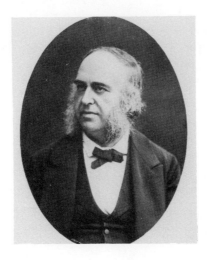

BROCA was not the first to put forward the hypothesis of cerebral localisation. Various people had thought on similar lines, and especially Boillaud who in 1825, concluded from clinico-pathological studies that loss of speech was associated with a lesion in a frontal lobe. This observation lay fallow for a generation until Broca described a case of a 51-year-old man, named Laborgue, who had lost his faculty of speech at the age of 30. His only utterance was the monosyllable, "Tan", repeated twice. "Tan" became his nickname. Ten years later paralysis of the right arm and leg slowly developed.

"Tan" died on 7th April 1861 and his brain was examined. There was degeneration of the cortex of the third left convolution which extended to the striate body producing hemiplegia. Broca called the loss of speech aphemia and it was Trousseau who suggested the name aphasia. Pierre Marie, who examined "Tan's" brain, emphasised that damage was extensive in the temporal and

17

parietal areas and attributed the aphasia to loss of intellectual capacity.

Broca supported Marie's theory later when, in 1864, he wrote a paper entitled, "Deux cas d'aphemie traumatique produite par des lesions de la troisième circonvolution frontal gauche" (Bull. Soc. Chir. Paris 1864 5 51). The "circonvolution du langage", or left inferior frontal gyrus, was named Broca's convolution by David Ferrier (1843-1928).

Broca was born on 28th June 1824 at Sainte-Foy-la-Grande, near Bordeaux, the son of a country practitioner of Huguenot stock. Having a great capacity for hard work and a prodigious memory, he took his bachelor's degree with high honours at the age of 16 in the Faculty of Literature and Science of the College of Sainte Foy, a popular seat of learning with the protestant youth of France. The death of his only sister caused him to alter his original plan for a military career and, with the support of his father, he entered the Faculty of Medicine in Paris in 1841. Here prizes and appointments fell into his lap. He received the degree of M.D. in 1849 and later won the title, Surgeon of the Hospitals, and became professor of surgery. He died suddenly of cardiac infarction on 8th July, aged 56, when at the height of his powers.

Although Broca's best known contribution to scientific knowledge was his hypothesis of cerebral localisation he was a great worker in the field of anthropology. The first anthropological society in France was founded under his aegis in 1861 and, as it was thought to have political aspirations, the special police used to attend its meetings. In 1872 Broca founded the Review of Anthropology. A prolific writer, he had over 500 publications of which a contemporary said: "He never wrote anything mediocre".

Broca was a heavily built man of rather fiery temperament but benevolent. He was adored by his associates. He married the wealthy daughter of J. G. Lugol, of Lugol's iodine fame. He received two of France's highest honours — membership of the French Academy of Science and, in the year of his death, membership of the Senate of the French Republic representing "France et Science".

Names We Remember

Although we now know that the functions of the cerebral cortex are not determined by well-defined areas and that cortical changes in aphasia are not limited to Broca's area, the name of Broca will remind us of the basic work he did on the physiology of speech.

BRUCELLOSIS
Sir David Bruce 1855-1931

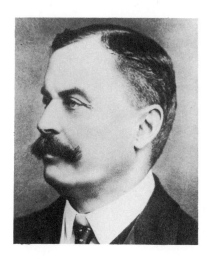

EVERYONE in Malta knew at the end of the last century that there was an illness there affecting many of the population with bouts of fever and general ill-health. It occurred in other Mediterranean countries also and was called Cyprus fever and Gibraltar fever as well as Malta fever. But the cause was unknown until David Bruce, who had been commissioned in 1853 in the Army Medical Service, was posted to Malta in 1886. After two years' work Bruce cultured a micrococcus from the spleens of fatal cases. He called it *Micrococcus melitensis* after the ancient name for Malta but since 1920 it has been called *Brucella melitensis* in honour of him. It was a remarkable discovery for a man without special training in microbiology. Subsequent investigation by a Royal Commission showed that 40 per cent of the island's goats were infected and 2,000 were excreting the organism in their milk. Prohibition of the use of goat's milk led to a dramatic fall in the incidence of Malta fever.

Bruce's approach to Malta fever and other medical problems was a biological one. After Malta his next tour of duty was to South Africa. The Governor of Natal, Sir Walter Hely-Hutchinson, already knew of Bruce's work in Malta and persuaded the army authorities to second him to work on a cattle disease, nagana, which was causing heavy losses. Within a few weeks Bruce had found a trypanosome (now called *Trypanosoma brucei*) in the blood of sick animals and showed that it was transmitted by a tsetse fly. His conquest of the cattle plague made the farmers refer to him as Bruce of Natal.

Another disease which Bruce conquered was sleeping sickness, or nergo lethargy. Aldo Castellani had noted a trypanosome in the cerebro-spinal fluid of patients with the disease but it was left to Bruce to complete the story. He found trypanosomes in the blood and, prompted by his earlier studies of nagana, he showed that they were carried by a tsetse fly.

David Bruce was an Australian of Scottish ancestry, born in Melbourne, Victoria, on 29th May 1855. His father had gone there in the gold rush to install a crushing mill. The family returned to Scotland when David was five and he received his early education at Stirling High School. Leaving at 14, he was employed in a business in Manchester but this job did not last long. His boyhood interest in natural history, and especially ornithology, led to his original intention to pursue zoology but in the end he chose medicine. He became a medical student in Edinburgh in 1876. Graduation in 1881 was followed by a short period of private practice in Reigate where, in 1883, he married Mary Elizabeth Steele, the daughter of his chief's predecessor.

Bruce was a man of fine physique and, but for an attack of pneumonia in his youth, he might have made athletics his career. Rather reserved in manner and very downright in speech, he often expressed himself forcibly and with shrewd wit. He was most straightforward and absolutely loyal to his fellow workers. His discoveries were of the greatest importance at a time when many advances were being made in the field of tropical medicine. He received many honours including the F.R.S. and a knighthood. Lady Bruce accompanied her husband everywhere, including the seige of Ladysmith, and as well as looking after him became skilled in all the techniques of his work. He never ceased to stress the part she played and said his discoveries could not have been made without her. When she died after a long illness he was too overcome by grief to attend the funeral and actually died himself during the funeral service.

BUERGER'S DISEASE
Leo Buerger 1879-1943

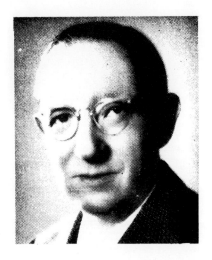

BUERGER'S disease is characterised by inflammation and thrombosis of both arteries and the veins, usually in the legs. Leo Buerger gave his original description of it in The American Journal of the Medical Sciences in 1908 (136 567). His article was entitled, "Thrombo-angiitis obliterans: a study of the vascular lesions leading to pre-senile spontaneous gangrene".

"The disease", wrote Buerger,
"occurs frequently, although not exclusively, among the Polish and Russian Jews, and it is in the dispensaries and hospitals of New York City that we find a good opportunity for studying it in its two phases, namely, in the period which precedes and in that which follows the onset of gangrene. We usually find it occurring in young adults between the ages of twenty and thirty-five or forty years ... After longer or shorter periods, characterised by pain, coldness of the feet, ischaemia, intermittent claudication and erythromelalgic symptoms,

23

evidence of trophic disturbances appear which finally pass over into a condition of dry gangrene . . . I . . . have come to the conclusion that we are dealing here with a thrombotic process in the arteries and veins followed by organisation and canalisation and not with an obliterating endarteritis . . . I would suggest that the name "endarteritis obliterans" and "arteriosclerotic gangrene" be discarded in this connection and that we adopt the term "obliterating thrombo-angiitis" of the lower extremities when we wish to speak of the disease under discussion'.

Buerger began collecting material in 1908 and some years later was able to report on a study of 40 amputated limbs, two amputated forearms and 25 extirpated veins from 18 patients with thrombo-angiitis afflicted with migrating phlebitis of the superficial veins. He thought the condition had an infective cause but attempts to demonstrate this have never been conclusive and present opinion places the condition among the collagen disorders.

Leo Buerger was born in Vienna on 13th September 1870 but came to the U.S.A. when one year old. Little is known of his childhood. He was educated at the College of the City of New York, at Columbia University and at the College of Physicians and Surgeons. He obtained the degrees of M.A. and M.D. in 1901. After acting for three years as a surgical intern at the Lennox Hill Hospital he served as a voluntary assistant at the Breslau Surgical Clinic in Germany, returning to private practice in New York in 1906. He was attached to the famous Mount Sinai Hospital for many years as a surgical pathologist. In the field of urology he had early recognised the need for an improved cystoscope and in 1909 brought out his perfected instrument on which F. Tilden Brown also worked (The Brown-Buerger cystoscope).

Buerger was a short dapper man, immacutely groomed and with expensive tastes in motor cars. He had a lifelong interest in music and his first wife, from whom he was divorced, was a concert pianist. After remarriage in 1929 he migrated to Los Angeles to be professor of urology at the College of Medical Evangelists.

Buerger was an egotist and it is said that he tried to have the name of Brown removed from the Brown-Buerger cystoscope. He was not well received in California where he announced that he had come to Los Angeles to teach local urologists how to practise urology. When he returned to New York in 1934 he was not taken back on the staff at Mount Sinai and had to be content with posts at a number of small private hospitals.

As well as making important endoscopic innovations Buerger broke new ground in many other aspects of surgery, working on shock and osteogenic sarcoma and in bacteriology. He wrote more than 120 medical articles and published a large monograph on the "Circulatory Disturbances of the Extremities".

Leo Buerger died in New York on 6th October 1943.

BURKITT'S LYMPHOMA
Denis Parsons Burkitt born 1911

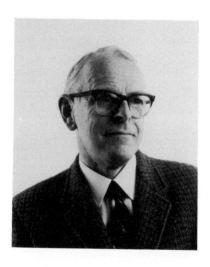

BURKITT's discovery of the tumour which bears his name followed a request made to him in 1957 by Dr Hugh Trowell, then senior physician at Mulago Hospital, Kampala, Uganda, to see a sick child called Africa. The child had swellings in all four quadrants of the jaws and Burkitt found it difficult to reconcile them with any known benign or malignant disease. He soon recognised other similar cases and found that nearly all had tumours in different parts of the body. What impressed him was that tumours in different sites, such as the jaws, orbits, ovaries, kidneys, liver, adrenals and thyroid, were associated, in different combinations, in the same patients. This observation convinced him that tumours in these diverse situations were not, as previously believed, different but were all manifestations of a single-tumour syndrome. This conviction was confirmed later by pathologists who showed that all the tumours were histologically identical.

When Dr George Oettlé, of the South African Institute for

Medical Research, on a visit to Kampala, said that such cases were never seen in South Africa Burkitt wondered why. In spite of much routine work he made many inquiries over the next three years about the incidence of such cases. He decided that to get the full story a personal search was necessary and so, with Dr Ted Williams and Dr Cliff Nelson, a 10,000-mile safari started which led them in six weeks to 57 hospitals in 12 countries. The object was to find out where the patients were living when the tumour first appeared.

The facts gleaned on this and other tours showed that the tumour occurred only in a belt of country across Africa which had a certain range of temperature and rainfall. The mechanism of the apparent height barrier which was first postulated really reflected temperature. The geographical distribution was very similar to that of several insect-vectored diseases including one, nyong nyong, known to be caused by an insect-borne virus. The circumstantial evidence suggested that Burkitt's lymphoma was similarly caused. At this stage it was called the "African lymphoma" but later it was found to occur also in Papua, New Guinea and Brazil where climatic conditions are similar. It is now known as a rare childhood tumour which can occur throughout the world but is common only where malaria is endemic. It is associated with antibodies to the Epstein-Barr virus but the etiology is more complicated than a straightforward virus infection and genetic factors may play a part also.

Burkitt first presented his work officially at the annual conference of the East African Association of Surgeons in January 1958 and published his first article later that year. It attracted little attention but, following another article, published in collaboration with Dr G. T. O'Conor in 1961, and lectures given in England, other workers began to realise the significance of Burkitt's epidemiological studies. Added interest arose when the tumour was shown to be remarkably sensitive to chemotherapy.

Denis Parsons Burkitt was born on 28th February 1911 at Enniskillen, near Lough Erne, in Northern Ireland. He began his education at Portora School in Enniskillen where he lost an eye after being hit by a stone. Later he attended a preparatory school in Anglesey and then went to a school in Cheltenham. He records that he was "poor to mediocre" at everthing except mathematics. At 18 he entered Dublin University to study engineering but had no enthusiasm for it. After a period of indecision he sought guidance in prayer and decided to become a medical student. Medicine thrilled him and five years later he graduated second in his class. His first post was a house surgeon in Chester. After that he spent six months at his teaching hospital in Dublin. Further posts in Preston and Poole were followed by study in Edinburgh where he became F.R.C.S. in 1958. A five-month trip as ship's surgeon in the "Glen Shiel", of the Blue Funnel Line, en route to Manchuria gave him time to think. He decided to work where medical need was much greater than in Europe and for further training he took a surgical post in Plymouth. The 1939-45 war had started but he was not then needed as a surgeon. He was turned down by the Colonial Office for service in Africa possibly because he had lost an eye. Later, however, he was accepted as a surgeon in the Armed Forces. In 1943, when on short leave, he married Olive Rogers who had been a nurse in Plymouth. A visit to Uganda during a posting to East Africa made him conscious of the medical needs of that country and when in 1946 he re-applied to join the Colonial Service he was accepted. Burkitt worked as a surgeon in Africa and became senior consultant at Mulago Hospital, Kampala, in 1961 and remained in Africa until 1966. Now as a member of the external staff of the Medical Research Council he continues his world-wide studies on disease distribution. His home is at Shiplake, Oxfordshire.

Geographical pathology is a rapidly expanding branch of medicine and for his work in this field he was elected F.R.S. in 1972. Burkitt would be the last man to seek eponymity and modestly gives credit for his discoveries to the qualities his parents gave him and the help of others.

Because the nature of the condition was then disputed, an International Cancer Congress in Paris in 1963 first adopted the eponym, "Burkitt's Tumour", but it is now universally recognised as lymphoma. Hence Burkitt, in his monograph; "Burkitt's Lymphoma", written with Dennis Wright and published in 1970, had no alternative but to adopt the eponymous name for it established by international usage.

BACILLE CALMETTE-GUÉRIN (BCG)
Léon Charles Albert Calmette 1863-1933
Jean-Marie Camille Guérin 1872-1961

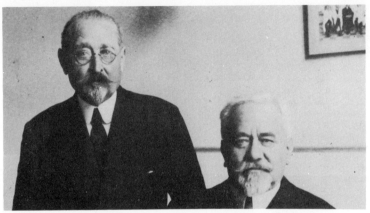

Guérin   Calmette

THE names of these two Frenchmen will always have a lasting place in the history of tuberculosis. The vaccine they discovered, known as BCG, is now used throughout the world under the sponsorship of the World Health Organisation and the United Nations Children's Emergency Fund.

ALBERT CALMETTE

Léon Charles Albert Calmette (known as Albert) was born at Nice on 12th July 1863 into a family of Breton origin. When a boarder at the Lycée at Brest ten of his colleagues died in a typhoid epidemic which impaired Calmette's own health and thwarted his ambition to become a sailor. So he entered the Naval Medical School at Brest and graduated at the University of Paris in 1886. After his first posting to the French Congo he was sent in 1889 to the islands of St Pierre and Miquelon, off Newfoundland, to work on the problem of red spots on salted cod which made it

29

unsaleable. Having shown that the spots were caused by a bacterium he found that a simple cure was to add sodium sulphite to the salt. He next worked in Saigon on snake venoms and produced a polyvalent serum. He also studied other infectious diseases including rabies. In 1895 he was sent by Pasteur to Lille to found the Lille Institute of Hygiene and there he worked for 25 years. The prevention of tuberculosis was his next task and it occupied him for the rest of his life.

Calmette was a cheerful, happy man who greatly inspired his students. He, like Pasteur, lived frugally and did not seek any material advantage. He was an indefatigible worker and when it was suggested that it would be wise for him to moderate his activity he replied: "J'espère qu'il me sera donné de travailler jusqu'a ce que mes yeux se ferment à la lumière et que je m'endormirai l'âme en paix avec la conscience d'avoir fait ce que j'ai pu".

On the death of Metchnikoff, Calmette became sub-director of the Pasteur Institute in Paris in 1917. He died on 29th October 1933 aged 70, after a few days' illness. The Lübeck disaster two years earlier had undermined his health though he lived to see his work vindicated.

CAMILLE GUÉRIN

Camille Guérin was born in Poitiers on 22nd December 1872. He used to accompany his father-in-law on his rounds as a veterinary surgeon and these visits made him decide to become a veterinarian himself. He attended the veterinary school at Alfort and was greatly impressed when Pasteur visited this school. After qualification as a veterinary surgeon he followed Calmette to Lille to be in charge of the laboratory of serums and vaccines. Always careful to avoid dispersion of his work, he concentrated all his activities on smallpox vaccination and tuberculosis. He was a scientist of scrupulous care and the strictest discipline. Always very punctual, he was at his laboratory half-an-hour before his colleagues. When he retired he continued to attend regularly the meetings at the Academy of Medicine. Apart from his academic knowledge he was often consulted because of his well-known commonsense approach in all matters.

Repeated subculture of an organism is known to cause loss of virulence. It is greatly to the credit of Calmette and Guérin that they continued subculturing for more than 12 years until they considered that, after 230 subcultures, the strain was irreversibly attenuated and incapable of causing tuberculosis. The bacilli were grown on potato soaked in bile. The crucial test of trials in man occurred in June 1921 when Dr Weill-Halle told Calmette about a tuberculous woman who had died after giving birth to a child. The grandmother who brought up the child was also tuberculous. In spite of constant exposure to tuberculosis, the child, who had been given BCG by mouth, did not develop the disease. Apart from the disaster at Lübeck, when 73 out of 250 infants vaccinated died of tuberculosis, there have been no untoward effects of BCG. (The disaster was due to carelessness in making the vaccine in the German laboratory).

CASTELLANI'S PAINT
Sir Aldo Castellani 1877-1971

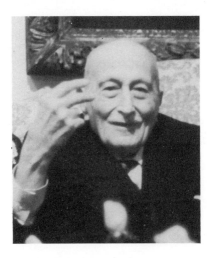

CASTELLANI'S name is remembered not so much for his eminence in international medicine as for the antiseptic paint he invented for the treatment of various skin diseases caused by fungi. It contains magenta, boric acid, phenol, resorscinol, acetone and alcohol and is described in the British Pharmacopoeial Codex as Magenta Paint.

Aldo Castellani was born on 8th September 1877, the youngest of three children of Italian parents who belonged to a distinguished Florentine family. He records that he adored his mother but had only filial respect for his father who imposed a very strict discipline. He always wanted to be a doctor although there were none among his forebears. Qualifying in 1899 at the age of 21 in the University of Florence he decided early to work in the tropics. So he came to London, being lured by the fame of Patrick Manson, the "father of tropical medicine" (see p. 92).

Manson recommended him as a member of the Royal Society's Commission on sleeping sickness and on 12th November 1903 he found a trypanosome in the cerebro-spinal fluid of a boy with the disease. He next went to Ceylon where he worked for 12 years as director of the Bacteriological Institute. It was here in 1905 that he discovered the spirochaete of yaws, now called *Treponema pertenue*. He said that his years in Ceylon were the happiest in his life.

In 1915 he returned to Italy as successor to Negri but was soon involved in the First World War in Serbia. Here he developed his technique of using a combined vaccine which, after initial opposition, was adopted by all the Allies although it did not bear out its pristine promise. As a mark of respect he was made professor of tropical medicine at Naples although at that time the city had no laboratory or hospital for tropical diseases.

In 1917 he became a member of the International Sanitary Commission and had the exceptional distinction of being a lieutenant-colonel in the Royal Italian Medical Service and an admiral in the Italian navy at the same time. In 1918 Castellani came back to London and when the Ross Institute was incorporated in the London School of Hygiene and Tropical Medicine he was made director of mycology. Perhaps his greatest interest lay in the fungi which caused skin diseases, until his day a virgin field.

He had now reached the height of his career. Although busy in London he took on the duties of professor of tropical medicine in Tulane University, New Orleans, to which he paid short visits for several years. He also worked in Paris. At the same time he edited the Journal of Tropical Medicine and Hygiene and conducted an enormous practice in Harley Street. It is recalled that on one occasion he had three European queens in his waiting room at the same time.

Because he had been surgeon-general in Mussolini's Ethiopian campaign he was deprived of his K.C.M.G. in 1940. This was restored to him a few weeks before he died. At the end of the war in Ethiopia King Victor Emanuel created him Count of Chisimaio and later raised him to the rank of Marchese.

Castellani was extremely loyal to his native land but almost equally an anglophile, although he never became a British subject. He was elected F.R.C.P. in 1922. In 1907 he married an Englishwoman, Josephine Ambler Stead, and had one daughter, Jacqueline, the present Lady Killearn. After the Second World War he left Italy for political reasons and settled in Cascais, Portugal, where he became medical adviser to the exiled Italian Royal family. Here he spent the remainder of his long life. He was made professor of pathology and tropical medicine at the Tropical Diseases Institute in Lisbon and so was able to continue his passionate devotion to tropical medicine and to keep his Jardin des Microbes which he had collected over the years. In 1960 he published his autobiography, "Microbes, Men and Monarchs". He was a prolific writer, mostly on dermatology, but some have felt that his later work did not maintain the standard of his earlier researches.

CHARCOT'S JOINTS
Jean-Martin Charcot 1825-1893

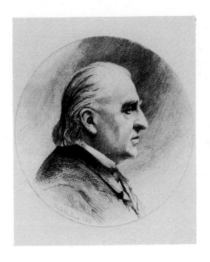

CHARCOT's name is kept alive in our memories chiefly as a convenient term for the painless arthropathy which occurs in tabes dorsalis. Similar joints are found in other conditions, such as syringomyelia, which interfere with the sensory pathways from joints. His story shows how he came to have such a prominent place among neurologists and physicians in the middle of the last century.

Jean-Martin Charcot was born in November 1825, the eldest of four sons of a Paris carriage-builder. He and his brothers were told that the one who received the best report from school would be entered for one of the learned professions. Jean-Martin was the winner and for a time his choice wavered between medicine and art. Selecting medicine, he began his studies in 1844 and qualified at the late age of 28. He was soon earning enough money to repay his parents. His career began and ended at the Hospice de la Salpêtrière, a vast museum of living pathology, so-called because at one time it was a gunpowder store of Louis XIII. In 1872 he became professor of pathological anatomy and in 1882 a chair of nervous diseases, the first of its kind in the world, was created for him.

Charcot had something of the artist in his make-up and it is not surprising that he made his clinic a world-famous show-place of clinical neurology. He had a huge amount of clinical material among the several thousand inmates upon whose nervous systems he could play as on a pipe in his dramatic twice-weekly lectures. These took place on a floodlit stage with Charcot standing beside his patient. The Tuesday clinics were impromptu affairs but on Fridays a lesson, prepared with the greatest care, was given on one subject. Eventually the demonstrations degenerated from scientific meetings to become sensational shows. As he had command of several languages, he attracted audiences from England, Germany, Spain and Italy. In private consultations his technique was to have an assistant who examined the patient first.

Charcot was the first to establish clinical neurology as a separate discipline and he unravelled more than one web of nerve pathology. As might be expected he was an inspiration to many pupils who became famous themselves, such as Marie, Babinski and Freud. In his hey-day his name was used eponymously for many neurological conditions for which we now have satisfactory descriptive terms. Amyotrophic lateral sclerosis, which he described in 1865, was known as the Maladie de Charcot but we now call it motor neurone disease. Peroneal muscular atrophy, which he wrote about in 1886, is still sometimes called Charcot-Marie-Tooth disease. He described cough syncope which he called "laryngeal vertigo". Charcot contributed to other branches of medicine as well as neurology. Rheumatoid arthritis is sometimes called Charcot's rheumatism on the Continent. In his thesis for his doctorate he distinguished between it and gout. Recurrent bouts of pyrexia in gallstone disease are sometimes referred to as Charcot's intermittent hepatic fever. In his clinical lectures on "Senile Diseases" (New Sydenham Society 1881) he called attention to the need for special study of the diseases of old age.

Charcot founded several medical journals such as the Archives of Experimental Medicine and Pathology and the Archives of

Neurology. His "Leçons sur les maladies du systeme faites à Là Salpêtrière" in 1872 saw many English translations. In later life Charcot became interested in hysteria. His views on it conflicted with those of some of his colleagues but he died before his radical revision of them was completed.

Charcot was smooth-shaven, of stocky build and medium height and is said to have resembled Napoleon, though Pierre Marie said his features were those of a Roman senator. He lived in great style in his palatial neo-Gothic home at 217 Boulevard Saint Germain in Paris. Here he was a generous host, his house being open on Tuesdays to all who wanted to come. His immense library had a two-storeyed gallery patterned after the medical library in the Convent of San Lorenzo at Florence. Charcot was careless of money and fees did not greatly interest him, for his wife was an heiress. His son, Jean Charcot (1867-1936) himself a neurologist, became a well-known explorer who died when his vessel, the Pourquoi-pas?, sank off Iceland with the loss of all hands.

In 1880 Charcot began to suffer from angina and he gave up work in 1893. He died in an attack of pulmonary oedema on the shore of the Lac des Lattons in the Morvan district on 16th August 1893. A statue in his memory stands in front of the Salpêtrière.

CHEYNE-STOKES BREATHING
John Cheyne 1777-1836

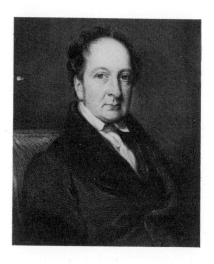

CHEYNE's name* would probably not have become eponymous
had not his paper on "A case of apoplexy in which the fleshy part
of the heart was converted into fat" (Dublin Hospital Reports
1818 2 216) been referred to by William Stokes (see p. 151) in his
famous book, "The Diseases of the Heart and Aorta", Dublin
1854, and in a paper in the Dublin Quarterly Journal of Medical
Sciences 1846

In describing periodic respiration Stokes says:
*'The symptom in question was observed by Dr Cheyne
although he did not connect it with the special lesion in the
heart. It consists in the occurrence of a series of inspirations,
increasing to a maximum and then declining in force and
length, until a state of apparent apnoea is established. In this*

---

*Not to be confused with a famous English physician, George Cheyne, author of
"An Essay of Health and Long Life".

condition the patient may remain for such a length of time as
to make his attendants believe that he is dead, when a low
inspiration followed by one more decided marks the
commencement of a new ascending and then descending
series of inspirations'.

As this account is not materially different from that of Cheyne, the current priority awarded to Cheyne in the eponym, Cheyne-Stokes respiration, seems proper. Cheyne's actual words in describing his patient's symptoms were:

" . . . for several days his breathing was irregular; it would
entirely cease for a quarter of a minute, then it would become
perceptible, though very low, then by degrees it became
heaving and quick and then it would gradually cease again".

John Cheyne, a Scotsman, was born at Leith on 3rd February, 1777 and had forbears in the medical profession. His father was a physician and his mother the daughter of William Edmonston, a Fellow of the Royal College of Surgeons of Edinburgh. At the Edinburgh High School he appears to have been unable to keep up with his class and he was therefore tutored at home by a clergyman, though without much progress. At the age of 12 he began to help his father with bleedings and dressings and was formally apprenticed to him at the age of 16. He seems to have absorbed a knowledge of medicine from this environment and, after coaching by a celebrated "grinder", Mr Caudlish, he qualified in 1795 at the age of 18. He entered the British Army in 1795 and served as an army surgeon for four years. He is said to have spent his time in "frivolous dissipation". On his return to Edinburgh he assisted his father and for some years had charge of an ordnance hospital at Leith. He worked with Mr (afterwards Sir) Charles Bell (see p. 11) and began to take the practice of medicine seriously. After a visit to Dublin in 1809 he decided at the age of 32 to practise there, "neither expecting, nor indeed wishing for, rapid advancement". In 1811 he became physician to the Meath Hospital and from then on his practice flourished and his income rose to £5,000 a year. He was the first professor of medicine at the Royal College of Surgeons of Ireland (1813) to which chair he was succeeded by Whitley Stokes, the father of William Stokes (see p. 151).

CONN'S SYNDROME
Jerome William Conn born 1907

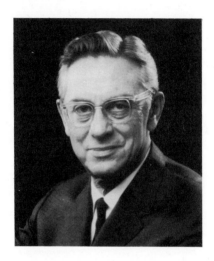

In 1944, during World War II, Dr Conn worked on the problem of
the acclimatisation mechanism involved when troops were
exposed to an unaccustomed hot, humid environment. He had
reported that there was increased production of a
"deoxycorticosterone-like" steroid and that this was reflected in
the sweat which had a very low sodium content. In 1954 he
encountered a 32-year-old woman patient whose muscular
weakness, large urinary volume and hypertension had been
attributed to kidney disease. But when the salt content of her sweat
was found to be very low the earlier studies were recalled and over-
production of a sodium-retaining steroid was suggested. Intensive
studies over a period of eight months supported this view and by
the time they were completed the hormone aldosterone had been
discovered in 1953 at the Middlesex Hospital, London, by Lawson
and Tait. Conn persuaded Dr William Baum to explore the
patient's adrenal glands. To everyone's delight, a cherry-sized

tumour was found in the right adrenal gland. It contained a very large amount of the new hormone. The patient was entirely cured of all her symptoms, including those of hypertension.

Conn's paper, "Primary Aldosteronism: a new clinical entity", written with L. H. Louis, appeared in the Transactions of the Association of American Physicians 1955 68 215. Pathologists sometimes refer to the cause as an aldosteronoma. Whether the popular label, Conn's syndrome, will survive remains to be seen, for the threat to the longevity of an eponym is the expanding knowledge of the disease it designates. Although the threat posed by the concept of pseudo-primary aldosteronism has been discounted the eponymity of Conn's syndrome may have been undermined. Nevertheless, the current use of his name justifies a few words about the remarkable man who made the initial discovery.

Jerome Conn was born in New York on 24th September 1907 of European parentage, his father being Austrian. At first, a business career was contemplated for him but as a schoolboy he built his crystal-set in an oatmeal box and it was clear that science fascinated him. He began his premedical studies at Rutger's University, New Jersey, in 1925 and graduated from the University of Michigan Medical School at Ann Arbor in 1932 at the age of 25. This has been his home ever since, for he met as a freshman a bright-eyed, attractive young medical student whom he married. After internships and residences he was drawn to the laboratory of Dr Louis Harry Newburgh, the first professor of clinical investigation at the University of Michigan Medical School at Ann Arbor. More than 30 years later he was awarded the distinguished (visiting) university professorship there in the name of Louis Harry Newburgh. Dr Conn became head of the department of endocrinology and metabolism and director of the Metabolism Research Unit, a post which he held until 1973. In 1974 he was made university professor emeritus at the University of Michigan and was appointed as the Veterans' Administration Distinguished Physician, only the seventh such appointment made in the U.S.A. He has laboratories at the Veterans' Administration Hospital in Ann Arbor. He has been president of the American Diabetes Association and is a member of the National Academy of Science of the U.S.A. and an honorary

41

member of numerous foreign professional societies. A fine esprit de corps exists in his team and he has refused tempting offers of posts in other places.

Dr Conn speaks with great clarity on complicated subjects and never uses notes. He watches his audience and can tell if they are not following him. In this way he can circle back and pick up the stragglers who have missed a point in his presentation. He is a prolific writer, with well over 300 papers in the field of metabolism. The massive amount of current world medical scientific literature has made him adopt a combined desk and work table 30 feet long. The saga of this physician in academic medicine is well described in his address for the general reader, "Blood, sweat, tears — and other biological fluids", published in the Michigan Alumnus Quarterly Review 1961 66 21. A heart attack in 1955 slowed him down a bit, but only temporarily, and he remains active in the field of medical research. Now at the age of 70 he still plays a reasonable game of tennis. His almost life-long enthusiasm for sport was probably instituted by his mother who gave him a baseball bat when he was nine.

CROHN'S DISEASE
Burrill Bernard Crohn born 1884

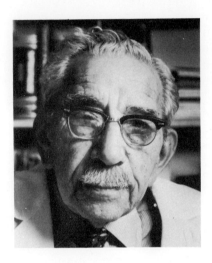

It is not often that a medical audience hears the announcement of a "new" disease, but this privilege was enjoyed by the members of the section of gastroenterology and proctology of the American Medical Association assembled for their 83rd annual meeting at New Orleans on 13th May 1932. On that day Drs Burrill B. Crohn, Leon Ginzburg and Gordon D. Oppenheimer read a paper entitled "Regional enteritis: a pathologic and clinical entity". Two years earlier Dr Crohn had persuaded Dr A. A. Berg to operate on a youth of 17 who had an abdominal mass, diarrhoea, abdominal pain and pyrexia. Tests for tuberculosis were negative and resection was successful. This and 13 similar cases formed the basis of the paper which was published in the Journal of the American Medical Association 1932 99 ii 1323-1329, but Berg modestly declined to add his name to it.

Dr Crohn and his associates stated that they proposed
"to describe in its pathological and clinical details a disease of

the terminal ileum affecting mainly young adults, characterised by subacute or chronic necrotising and cicatrising inflammation. The ulceration of the mucosa is accompanied by a disproportionate connective tissue reaction of the remaining walls of the involved intestine, a process which frequently leads to stenosis of the lumen of the intestine associated with the formation of multiple fistulas. The disease is clinically featured by symptoms that resemble those of ulcerative colitis, namely fever, diarrhoea and emaciation leading eventually to an obstruction of the small intestine; the constant occurrence of a mass in the right iliac fossa usually requires surgical intervention (resection). The terminal ileum is alone involved".

In the discussion which followed the reading of the paper several of the older clinicians of wide experience said that they had seen such a condition in the past but had not known what to call it. The paper aroused tremendous interest and case reports began to pour in from all parts of the world under various titles such as "terminal ileitis", "chronic cicatrising enteritis" and "non-specific granuloma of the intestine". Crohn called it "terminal enteritis" but Bargen, of the Mayo Clinic, felt that "terminal" might be interpreted as meaning that death was imminent and his suggestion of "regional ileitis" was adopted. It was not long, however, before the eponymic name, Crohn's disease, was in universal use.

There is no doubt that isolated examples of what undoubtedly were cases of regional enteritis were reported long before Crohn's time. Morgagni may have written the first account of the disease in 1769. A paper was read on 4th July 1806 by Charles Combe (1743-1817), physician to the British Lying-in Hospital, on "a singular case of stricture or thickening of the ileum" (Medical Transactions of the College of Physicians, London, 1813 4 16). T. K. Dalziel wrote a paper in the British Medical Journal 1913 2 1068 entitled "Chronic Interstitial Enteritis", describing three cases which had undergone surgery. It seems probable that many cases diagnosed in the past as ileocaecal tuberculosis were in reality examples of Crohn's disease. Since 1932 Dr Crohn has published several notable articles on the condition. He has never made a claim to priority but he must certainly be given the credit for having published the first full and clear-cut clinical picture including the X-ray appearances, course and surgical treatment. Nothing has been subtracted from his original conception but much has been added. It is now known that the disease is not always limited to the terminal ileum and even the jejunum may be affected. Charles Wells, of Liverpool, in 1952 separated from ulcerative colitis cases of "segmental colitis" which he regarded as a colonic form of Crohn's disease.

Dr Crohn was born in New York City on 13th June 1884, the son of Theodore and Leah Crohn. He was educated at the College of the City of New York and at Columbia University and graduated in 1907. For his studies on the metabolism of gross haemorrhage he was offered the degrees of M.A. and Ph.D. but said he did not have the heart to ask his father for the fees. He was an intern at Mount Sinai Hospital for three-and-a-half years, being chosen by Dr Emanuel Libman, he says, because he had read German textbooks as well as Osler's. He was chief of the Gastroenterological Division of Mount Sinai Hospital from 1925 to 1969. His other appointments included those of consulting gastroenterologist to the Beth Israel Hospital. He enjoyed an international reputation as a gastroenterologist long before the appearance of his famous paper, largely because of his monograph on "Affections of the Stomach" (1927) and his other writings. He was president of the American Gastroenterological Association in 1932. Dr Crohn is now retired and lives in New York City.

CUSHING'S DISEASE
Harvey Williams Cushing 1869-1939

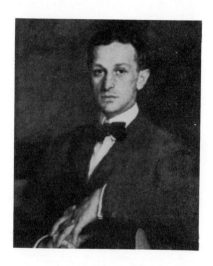

PLETHORIC adiposity with hypertension, muscle wasting, skin striae and osteoporosis are the clinical features of what used to be called Cushing's syndrome — a rare condition. Cushing's first case (Bulletin of the Johns Hopkins Hospital 1932 50 137) had a basophil adenoma of the pituitary. As the mechanism is now known to be excess production of adrenocorticotrophic hormone (A.C.T.H.), modern physicians use the term Cushing's disease or pituitary-dependent adrenal hyperplasia. A similar non-pituitary-dependent picture is produced by cortisol-secreting adrenal neoplasms and by ectopic production of A.C.T.H. by neoplasms such as bronchial carcinoma. Excessive corticosteroid therapy can result in a similar picture.

Harvey Cushing was born in Cleveland, Ohio, on 8th April 1869, being the ninth child in a sibship of ten of Henry Kirke and Betsy Marie Cushing. A forbear, Matthew Cushing, had settled in Hingham in the Massachussets Bay colony, having come to

U.S.A. in the Diligent, arriving in Boston on 10th August 1638. Cushing's immediate ancestors were eminent in medicine, Harvey being the fourth in line to practise. His father was professor of obstetrics and gynaecology in the Western Reserve University School of Medicine. Harvey first went to Yale and studied under R. H. Chittenden, the physiological chemist. In his final year he became interested in medicine and, after graduating in 1891, he went to Harvard and graduated in medicine there in 1895. After interning at the Massachussets General Hospital he entered the surgical service of Halsted, in Baltimore, in 1896. While still a student he and a colleague, E. A. Codman, devised ether charts which were used to record the pulse, respiration etc. during operations. Next followed a period of travel abroad in the company of William Osler and Thomas McCrae, both of whom later also became world-famous. Cushing worked in France, Switzerland, Italy and England where, with Sherrington, he studied the motor cortex in anthropoids.

Cushing's experience abroad made him decide to develop brain surgery and he pursued his aim with great determination. He learned surgical technique from Halsted at the Johns Hopkins Hospital, Baltimore, and clinical neurology from Osler. On his return to Boston in 1891 he began his practice as a neurosurgeon and developed a precise technique which often achieved success where failure had been the rule. His colleagues were against the attempted removal of intra-cranial tumours but Cushing's enthusiasm received great impetus from his successful removal of a large meningioma from the chief-of-staff of the U.S. Army who returned to duty within a month and continued in good health for 17 years. As well as perfecting his operative skill, Cushing made fundamental contributions to our knowledge of the physiology of the brain and cerebro-spinal fluid though some of his conclusions about pituitary endocrine functions were later proved wrong.

In 1902, when aged 43, he was Moseley professor of surgery at Harvard and surgeon-in-chief to the Peter Bent Brigham Hospital, Boston. He favoured private practice and so always advocated part-time, as opposed to full-time, clinical professorships. Neurosurgery had long been a mere adjunct to general surgery but Cushing raised it to the status of a recognised speciality. As early as 1904 he read a paper to the Cleveland

Academy of Medicine entitled "The Special Field of Neurological Surgery". In 1911 he founded the Society of Neurological Surgeons. In the First World War Cushing helped to organise a Harvard surgical unit (The American Ambulance) and served with it in France for several months before American entry into the war. He went to France in May 1917 and did brilliant work as an army surgeon, becoming the senior consultant in neurosurgery with the American Expeditionary Force. He received many military and civilian awards.

Cushing was a tall wiry man sharp features and a deep voice. He had great personal charm. Young surgeons flocked to him from all over the world. He practised an iron self-discipline, rising early and often doing much paper work before operating. At the end of an operation he dictated full notes of what he had done and often made beautiful sketches. While he was very kind and gentle with patients he could be a tyrant to nurses and students as he always demanded perfection. His temperament was stormy and there are stories of his clashes with others in the literary and military worlds. Later in life, Cushing became interested in medical history and made a complete collection of the works of Vesalius. He wrote a life of William Osler for which he received the Pulitzer Prize in 1925. An advocate of early retirement, he vacated his posts in Boston in 1932 and then spent his last seven years at Yale as Sterling professor of neurology and director of studies in the history of medicine.

Superlatives fail when we try to describe the professional career of this great man. He will go down in history as the one who first established scientific surgery of the brain. Cushing married Katherine Crowell in 1902 and they had three daughters and two sons. He died at New Haven on 7th October 1939 of coronary occlusion.

Note.

The Cushing chair of medicine at University College, Dublin, is named after Cardinal Cushing and not Harvey Cushing.

DARWINISM
DARWIN'S TUBERCLE
Charles Robert Darwin 1809-1882

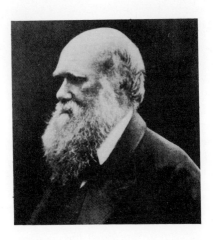

BEFORE Darwin's time the Church had dominated thinking on man's origin and supported the belief in a special six-day act of creation with subsequent fixity of all species. When this belief gave place to ideas of some kind of evolutionary process the problem was to explain the vast number of species known to exist. Charles Darwin's famous grandfather, Erasmus, had put forward the doctrine of inheritance of characteristics acquired because of a "desire" to change. Lamarck, a scientist (1744-1829), thought that one species grew out of another because of different use of certain organs called for by changes in the environment. These were only theoretical explanations and it was Charles Darwin who first convinced the world by evidence that evolution occurred because innate variations gave some members of a species an advantage which enabled them to prevail in the struggle for existence. This is Natural selection, popularly called "survival of the fittest", i.e. the most suitable to its environment and not necessarily the most physically vigorous.

The idea came to Darwin early but he did not want to build his theory entirely on fantasy and so repeat the mistake of his grandfather. He therefore postponed publication year after year but was always haunted by the dread that someone would forestall him. In 1848 a letter from Alfred Russel Wallace showed that he too, had independently formed the same theory. Fortunately, in 1844 Darwin, at a time when he thought he was dying, had written out his theory and sent it to Joseph Hooker and this letter established Darwin's priority. In 1848 Darwin and Wallace jointly presented to the Linnean Society of London the theory of evolution by natural selection. "The Origin of Species" was completed in November 1859. It met with immediate success, the first edition of 1,250 copies being sold out on the day of publication.

Charles Robert Darwin was born on 12th February 1809 at The Mount, Shrewsbury, the fifth of the six children of Robert Waring Darwin, a medical practitioner. His mother, Susanna Wedgwood, daughter of the great potter, died when he was young and he was brought up entirely by his rather autocratic father who placed him and his brother as medical students in Edinburgh. Charles thought anatomy disgusting and refused to dissect though he later regretted this. When he summoned the courage to tell his father this he was allowed to transfer to Christ's College, Cambridge, with a view to entering the Church. He was an unremarkable student who enjoyed the non-scholastic activities and said himself that he was lucky to get a pass degree. Charles was always interested in natural history and the collection of insects. He was fond of doing experiments and his school friends had called him "gas". When the offer came of an unpaid post of natural history expert on an Admiralty barque, H.M.S. Beagle (Captain Robert Fitzroy), which was to survey the coast of South America, Darwin was very interested. His father was against his application but agreed that if one person could be found to support it he would not object. Darwin's philosopher and reformer uncle, Josiah Wedgwood, wrote to Dr Robert Darwin in support and opposition was withdrawn.

The Beagle was a "coffin ship" (so-called because of its rotten timber), 90 feet long and of 242 tons, and sailed from Plymouth on 27th December 1831 with a company of 74. She returned on 2nd

October 1835 after a voyage lasting five years. What Darwin saw in the Galapagos Islands made them the birthplace of his theory and it was quite clear by then that he would never become a clergyman. A year after his return he was married at the age of 30 to his favourite cousin, Emma Wedgwood, on 29th January 1839, and settled in the Kentish town of Downe. Here, in Down House, he gradually became a nervous invalid and a recluse. He wrote: "I never pass 24 hours without having hours of discomfort". He never travelled abroad again and died in 1882 at the age of 73.

Much has been written about Darwin's illness. The general conclusion is that it was an inherited form of depression or a neurosis which provided him with the leisure to pursue his studies and protected him from the chores of life. The theory that it was due to infection with a trypanosome (Chagas' disease) contracted in South America remains unproved. Darwin was determined not to let his health interfere with what he wanted to do and so he avoided seeing a doctor before the Beagle sailed lest he might have been prevented from going.

Down House was large, cold, draughty, without a bathroom and "of surpassing ugliness". Darwin worked in a small room on the ground floor with a writing board on his knees in a chair which his grandfather had used. Here he carefully arranged his notes on bits of paper to build up his theory. He would breakfast alone at 7.45 a.m. and then work for short periods with frequent breaks for a walk round the garden. The vigorous young man who sailed the world in The Beagle became the chronic invalid who lived "the life of the shawl".

Darwin has been called "the Newton of Biology" but he was not clever in the popular sense. He wrote that he was "always a slow thinker, lacking the wit of many in conversation". His memory was poor and he was never able to remember for more than a few days a single date or line of poetry. But he liked work and did it for the sheer joy of investigation. He had no sense of humour and his leg was pulled when he included in the first edition of the Origin of Species the story of a bear swimming with its mouth open to skim off insects in the water. He said he saw no reason why a race of bears should not arise with large mouths like whales. The edition was withdrawn when he learned that the story was just a practical joke. Darwin's idea of evolution was not original, but he provided the facts on which its true mechanism is based and made it not only probable but inescapable. Based as it was on the thesis of man's rise by natural selection it was much attacked by theologians who preferred the idea of man's fall from God's grace.

Darwin's last piece of research ended years of patient observation of the common earthworm. He showed that particles of chalk put on his lawn became deeper and deeper over the years as the worms brought up earth to the surface.

Eponymity in Darwin's case comes not only in the term Darwinism, by which his theory of evolution is known, but also on account of an anatomical deformity of the ear (Darwin's ear). The helix is absent at the upper and outer part so that the free border forms a sharp point upwards and outwards. Sometimes a blunt point projects from the upper part of the ear (Darwin's tubercle). Darwin's attention was drawn to this by Woolner, the sculptor, and it is sometimes called Woolner's tip.

Although no official honour was awarded to him during life Darwin was accorded burial in Westminster Abbey. Down House was taken over by the Royal College of Surgeons and restored with the help of his sixth child, Major Leonard Darwin.

DUPUYTREN'S CONTRACTURE
Guillaume Dupuytren 1777-1835

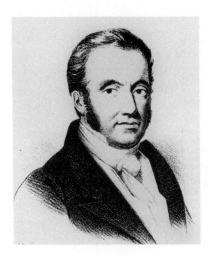

IT is given to few to rise from real poverty to great riches and become physician to kings. Yet this briefly is the story of Guillaume Dupuytren. He was born in 1777 at Pierre-Buffière, near Limoges, in Central France, where his father was a struggling solicitor. At the age of four he was so attractive that he was kidnapped by a wealthy lady and taken to Toulouse. After restoration to his parents another rich person, a cavalry officer, fell victim to his charms and arranged to pay for his education in Paris. Guillaume wanted a military career but his father, reminding him of the many surgeons there had been in the Dupuytren family, commanded: "Tu seras chirurgien". When Guillaume started his medical studies he was practically penniless. He lived in the cheapest room on a diet of bread and cheese and is said to have used the fat from bodies in the dissecting room for his lamp. Yet he overcame these handicaps for to him an obstacle was simply something to be surmounted.

In 1802, at the age of 25, he was elected to the post of surgeon of the second class at the Hôtel-Dieu after the usual concours or trial of ability. He became surgeon-in-chief eleven years later, a post he had always coveted, and had the use of 100 of the 250 beds. He had qualified in 1802 but could not take his degree until 1803 as the medical schools were closed temporarily by the revolutionary government.

Dupuytren worked at the Hôtel-Dieu for 33 years. Throughout this period he had superabundant energy. He would arrive to make rounds at 6 a.m. wearing his green coat, white waistcoat, blue trousers and a green cloth cap. After mammoth operating sessions he made more rounds in the evening. He insisted on doing everything himself and left little to his assistants, pursuing his work with almost religious dedication. He seemed to delight in finding fault with his staff and his assistants hardly opened their mouths in his presence. Only his child patients were exempt from his rudeness. A nervous habit which he showed constantly was to gnaw the nails of his left thumb and index finger.

The main operations of those days were amputations following fractures, the removal of bladder stones and the relief of strangulated hernias. But this fearless and brilliant operator carried out with the greatest skill other procedures such as excision of the lower jaw, ligation of the subclavain artery and the making of a lumbar colostomy. Even so he regarded an operation as "an evil alternative which nothing short of positive necessity should induce the surgeon to adopt". His practice was large and lucrative. He was a first-class orator and had few peers in Europe as a teacher. His inspiring lectures were always crowded. They often continued as he walked from the hospital. "Read little, see much, do much" was his advice to students. All recognised his pre-eminence, and his self-confidence was expressed in his own words: "I have been mistaken but I have been mistaken less than other surgeons". He was held in awe and even disliked by many of his contemporaries who referred to him as "The brigand of the Hôtel-Dieu". That Dupuytren's reputation was mixed is shown by the epigram, "First among surgeons, last among men". He was also called "the Napoleon of surgery" and he certainly reigned alone at the Hôtel-Dieu. In addition to his supreme skill he had a marked capacity for self-advancement or savoir-vivre which aroused antagonism in his contemporaries. Laennec, for example, broke with him and set up his own separate school of pathology.

Dupuytren was an atheist with an innate paranoid tendency and, after his wife deserted him, he became more cynical and distrustful. The surgeon in Honoré de Balzac's story "La Messe de l'Athée" is clearly Dupuytren. Mediocrity was his greatest fear. "Nothing should be feared so much for a man as mediocrity", he said.

Dupuytren became surgeon to Charles X and Louis XVIII though his atheism almost prevented these appointments. When he was created a baron only his intimates were allowed to call him "Le Baron". When Charles X became financially embarrassed Dupuytren wrote to him: "Sire, Grace in part to your benefactions I possess three millions. I offer you one; I intend the second for my daughter and the third I reserve for my old age". The King declined this beau geste.

Intending to retire at 60, Dupuytren unfortunately had a stroke in November 1833 when walking to the Hôtel-Dieu and had to give up work. Advised to rest he replied: "Le repos, c'est la mort" ("Rest, that's death"), and he died on February 8th 1835, aged 57, while his doctors were debating whether to drain his empyaema. "It is better" he said, "to die of the disease than of the operation". Despite his rise from poverty to affluence, or perhaps because of it, he had remained a parsimonious and cold man. His brusque manner did not make friendship easy and it has been said of him that he was a man "whom all admired, few loved and none understood".

What we now call Dupuytren's contracture had been recognised earlier by Astley Cooper (1768-1841) in England and Boyer in France. However, Dupuytren's description of the condition in the first volume of his Leçons Orales in 1832 and his demonstration that the disability of the ring and little fingers arose from a lesion of the aponeurosis, and not of the skin or tendons justify the eponym. In 1831, after dissecting the hand of a cadaver with the condition, he divided the aponeurosis in a coachman whose contracture was attributed to holding his whip too tightly. The basic cause is now known to be metabolic. Dupuytren made numerous other contributions to surgery and he would probably have been piqued that posterity has ignored them. He hated to write and left his surgical records largely to his students though he revised their work.

FALLOT'S TETRALOGY
Etienne-Louis Arthur Fallot 1850-1911

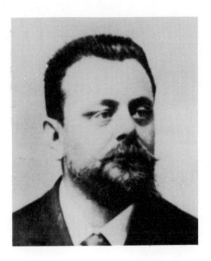

AN early description of the abnormalities in the "blue baby" as found in a post-mortem examination on a fetal monster was given by Niels Stensen (1628-1686), the Danish anatomist who discovered the parotid duct. They were also mentioned by a Dutch physician, Edward Sandifort (1742-1814), as the necropsy findings in a blue boy. But it was Fallot who correlated the clinical and pathological findings in his description of the maladie bleue, based on the findings in two patients under his care and a study of 50 others in the literature.

Fallot's paper, "Contribution a l'anatomie pathologique de la maladie bleue", was published in an obscure journal, Marseille-médical 1888 25 418. In it he said: "This malformation consists of a true anatamo-pathologic type represented by the following tetralogy: stenosis of the pulmonary artery, interventricular communication, deviation of the origin of the aorta to the right and hypertrophy, almost always concentric, of the right ventricle.

Failure of obliteration of the foramen ovale may occasionally be added in a wholly accessory manner". He showed that the cyanosis and other features may not appear during the first years of life and that some of the patients had lived for more than 60 years.

Arthur Fallot was born at Cette (Sète) on the Mediterranean coast of France on 29th September 1850. Because, at his request, no obituary was written on his death little is known of his life. He is said to have shown high scholastic ability at the Lycée in Marseilles. He became a medical student at nearby Montpellier in 1867. He was an intern in Marseilles where in 1876 he was granted the degree of M.D. for a thesis on pneumothorax. He had a busy practice and in 1888 he was appointed professor of hygiene and legal medicine at Marseilles. He died on 30th April 1911.

HANSEN'S BACILLUS
Gerhard Henrik Armauer Hansen 1841-1912

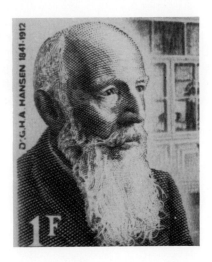

LEPROSY was common in the Bergen area of Norway in the 1880s. It had been on the decline but the resulting opening of the leprosy hospital to non-lepers caused the incidence to increase. More accommodation for lepers was needed and in 1849 the Lungegaard Hospital was opened in Bergen with Daniel Cornelius Danielssen, "the father of leprosy", in charge. He thought that the disease was inherited and Hansen was to prove him wrong by his discovery of the bacillus of leprosy.

Armauer Hansen was born in Bergen on 29th July 1841, the eighth child in a family of 15 of a well-to-do merchant. He was a very serious and earnest young man, interested in natural history and an eager defender of Darwin's theory (see p. 59). He worked for a time in a girls' school and as an overt agnostic he expressed concern over the religious teaching to which he was exposed. He qualified at the University of Christiania, (now Oslo), in 1866. After a year as an intern and a few months as physician in the

Lofoten Islands he became assistant physician to the Lungegaard Hospital in 1868. He was offered the chance to work in pathology at Bonn but Germany was at war with France at the time and so he went to Vienna instead. He returned to Bergen in 1871 and, though at first he felt revulsion for leprosy, this soon gave place to fascination, and from then on he became a life-long student of it.

The idea that a living micro-organism could cause disease had few supporters at that time and Hansen did not publicise his discovery of "small staff-like bodies much resembling bacteria". One reason for his reluctance to proclaim his work was that he did not wish to be in conflict with Danielssen with whose daughter, Stephanie, he was in love. He married her in January 1873 when he was 32 and she 27. She died of tuberculosis in October of the same year. (Hansen married again in 1875 and had one son whom he called Daniel Cornelius, after his mentor).

The date of Hansen's discovery is usually given as 28th February 1873 and he communicated his observation on the etiology of leprosy to the Medical Society of Christiania in 1874, but he first saw the bacteria in 1869 in biopsy material from a leprous nodule. In 1879 Professor Neisser of Breslau went to Bergen and studied Hansen's material. He took some of it back to Germany where he succeeded in staining the bacilli. This led him to claim the discovery of them for himself and the Germans spoke of the bacillus of Neisser. Danielssen scolded his son-in-law for letting someone steal his discovery and for a time a compromise name, the Hansen-Neisser bacillus, was used. Later, when Hansen published his observations it became known as Hansen's bacillus.

As well as discovering the bacillus of leprosy Hansen did great work in the management of the disease. For example, he caused the Norwegian custom of "laegd" to be abolished. In this, poor lepers were provided for by sending them from farm to farm to work for a few weeks. The abandonment of this practice and the introduction of other measures caused the incidence of the disease to fall from 2,833 cases in 1850 to only 140 in 1923.

Hansen's bacillus has not yet fulfilled all of Koch's postulates and it is doubtful even now whether transmission has ever been achieved, except perhaps in the armadillo. An attempt to transmit the disease by injecting material into the eye of a patient, although unsuccessful, led to a court action which cost Hansen his job. He was prohibited from practising in hospital for the rest of his life. But he remained official adviser to the Government and occupied a prominent position among the physicians of his time. In 1901 he was given the highest possible salary as a reward.

Hansen died on 12th February 1912 when on an official journey to the little town of Floro where he was found dead one morning, having been "glad and contented" the previous day. He had had symptoms of coronary ischaemia for some time. He was accorded a state funeral. A bust in the Pleistiftelsen für Spedalske in Bergen shows his striking appearance and his sharp and pronounced nose.

THE HARVEIAN SOCIETY
THE HARVEIAN ORATION
William Harvey 1578-1657

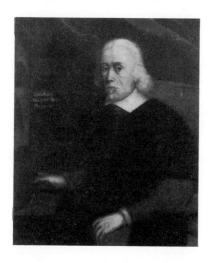

THERE are quibbles about various early anatomical accounts suggesting that the blood circulated in the body but Harvey's was the correct one. It is as its discoverer and as creator of quantitative experimental physiology that his place in the history of medicine is secure. But as there is no disease, test, sign or instrument connected eponymously with his name its inclusion here must rest on the societies and commemorative functions named after him. A very great deal has been written about Harvey as a clinician and scientist and all that is intended now is to record briefly the facts about his life.

Harvey was born at Folkestone on 1st April 1578, the eldest of the seven sons of Thomas Harvey who was Mayor of Folkestone in 1600. His father clearly intended him for learning rather than trade and so William entered The King's School, Canterbury, in 1588. He matriculated as an ordinary student at Gonville and

Caius College at the age of 15. The medical curriculum at Cambridge at the time was mediocre and Harvey was able to take advantage of the Matthew Parker scholarship in 1593 (£3 0s 8d for 6 years and lodging "for able, learned and worthy youths born in Kent and educated at Canterbury") and go to Padua where he graduated M.D. with high honours on 25th April 1602.

On his return to London he lived in Ludgate. He was married on 24th October 1604 when he was 26 to Elizabeth Browne, the daughter of Lancelot Browne, a doctor of physic. They had no children. Five years later he was made F.R.C.P. and shortly afterwards became physician to St Bartholomew's Hospital. He was also attached to the Court, being appointed physician-in-ordinary to the King at a salary of £300 per annum. He served first King James I (1566-1625) and then King Charles I (1600-1649) with whom he was intimate. The animals in the royal parks were put at Harvey's disposal and King Charles was greatly interested in the studies Harvey made on them. Harvey was orthodox in religion and politics but not in his ideas about the heart which were revolutionary. In the Civil War parliamentary troops ransacked his house in Whitehall and many of his clinical and anatomical records were destroyed. Harvey spent the years 1640 to 1642 in Oxford as warden of Merton College, a post to which the King had appointed him.

At the end of his life, a childless widower, with his post at St Bartholomew's Hospital ended, he busied himself with the affairs of the Royal College of Physicians. He was both a censor and an elect though he had to refuse the presidency on grounds of health (he suffered from gout). He died on 3rd June 1657 of cerebral haemorrhage at the house of his brother, Eliab, at Roehampton, and was buried uncoffined but "lapped in lead" at Hempstead, near Saffron Walden, Essex, where there is a marble mausoleum. A marble bust and several portraits in oils are at the Royal College of Physicians of London and there is a bust in the great hall at St Bartholomew's Hospital. A large bronze statue is prominent on the Leas at Folkestone. It shows Harvey in his doctor's gown holding a heart in his left hand and feeling the beat of his own heart with his right hand. There is a memorial window in Folkestone Parish Church. The statue, which used to be in a niche over the entrance of the former house of the Royal College of

Physicians in Trafalgar Sqaure, London, is now to be seen in the garden of the William Harvey public house at Willesborough, near Ashford, Kent, on the site of a cottage where Harvey is said to have spent some of his childhood. Several small statuettes exist and there are replicas in many of the medical schools in Texas, donated on a visit by the members of the Harveian Society of London in 1972.

Harvey's friend, John Aubrey, described him as "not tall, but of the lowest stature, round-faced, olivaster complexion (like wainscot) little eye, round, very black, full of spirit; his hair was black as a Raven, but quite 20 years old before he dyed". He was rapid in speech and given to gesture.

Harvey's most famous work, Exercitatio Anatomica De Motu Cordis et Sanguinis in Animalibus, a little book of 72 pages, was published in Frankfurt in 1628. Unfortunately, because of the difficulty in interpreting Harvey's handwriting, it contained many errors. Harvey was the first to turn away from the speculation of Galen, saying: "The method of investigating truth commonly pursued at this time . . . is held to be erroneous and almost foolish, in which so many require what others have said and omit to ask whether the things themselves be actually so or not". An often quoted saying of Harvey is: "I avow myself the partisan of truth alone".

The Harveian Oration and feast have been held at the Royal College of Physicians of London almost without interruption since 1656. The West London Medical Society became the Harveian Society in 1831 and meets regularly. There is an Edinburgh Harveian Society and a Harvey Society of New York. No Harvey museum exists at present but it is hoped to bring one together, perhaps at Folkestone. There is a list of Harveian relics in the library of the Royal College of Physicians of London.

HASHIMOTO'S DISEASE
Hakaru Hashimoto 1881-1934

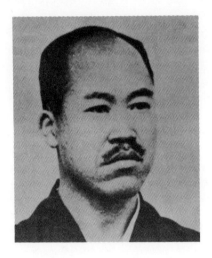

HASHIMOTO's lymphadenoid thyroiditis has been known since 1912 when Hashimoto published his paper on four cases of thyroid tumours in women aged between 40 and 61. He described his "struma lymphomatosa" in Archiv für Klinische Chirurgie 1912 7 219. The gland is enlarged and firm, from two to five times its normal size, and may be asymetrical and nodular. The thyroid parenchyma is atrophied so that thyroid function is diminished. It was not until 1956 that the patient's blood was shown to contain thyroid antibodies and the condition is now placed among the autoimmune disorders.

Hakaru Hashimoto, the third son of Kennosuke and Riyu Hashimoto, was born in the village of Midau, Nishi-tsuge, in the Mie prefecture, Japan, on 5th May 1881. He was the fifth of a line of medical practitioners and his grandfather was a very well-known doctor. After attending the Nishi-tsuge primary school in the village and other schools he entered the newly established medical school of Kyushu University in 1903. He is described as being a "diligent and taciturn" student with a quiet and unassuming manner. He was one of the founders of a students' association for cultural activities and a fervent Buddhist. In 1907 he was one of the first graduates in medicine from the University of Kyushu. He worked there from 1908 to 1912 in the surgical department under Professor Hauari Miyake to prepare his M.D. thesis on the then unknown condition, "Struma lymphomatosa". Few of his colleagues were aware of his discovery because his account of it was published in Germany.

After obtaining his M.D. he went to Europe, intending to spend three years in Berlin. Göttingen and London studying renal tuberculosis, but World War I caused him to return to Japan after two years. (A statement in an American journal that he lived in New York and was a Japanese American is incorrect). Because his father had died he went straight into the family practice and was soon a prosperous surgeon with a reputation in major abdominal surgery. He was a very hard worker but he often went to the theatre to see the traditional Japanese Kabuki play and was fond of eating out. He was careless about money and it is recorded that many of his patients did not pay their fees. Two further papers appeared, on erysipelas and on penetrating wounds of the chest wall. He died of typhoid on 9th January 1934 at the age of 52 (54 in the Japanese way of reckoning age). His grave is in the cemetery of Isshinzan Sennenji Temple, Midai, Iga-cho, Ayama-gun, Mie Prefecture. The words on the moss-covered headstone give his posthumous Buddhist name, Choshoin Reiyo Josho Sakushin Koji, which shows the great respect in which he was held. In 1937 Dr Hashimoto was honoured by the Physicians' Association of Ayama County in the Mie Prefecture who placed a bronze bust of him in front of the town hall of Iga-cho, the new name of Nishi-tsuge village. The hospital where he worked became in 1953 an old people's home, Kairaku-So, Iga-cho, Ayama-gun, Mie Prefecture.

HODGKIN'S DISEASE
Thomas Hodgkin 1798-1866

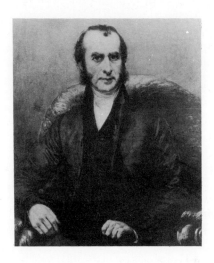

HODGKIN's first patient with the disease named after him was a ten-year-old boy, Ellenborough King, who was admitted to Guy's Hospital under the care of Dr Richard Bright. For 13 months he had enlargement of the neck glands and he also showed ascites and splenomegaly. Hodgkin collected six similar cases and gave an account of them in a paper entitled, "On some morbid appearances of the absorbent glands and spleen" (Medico-Chirurgical Transactions, 1832 17 68), and said:

> " . . . the enlargement of the glands appeared to be primary rather than the result of irritation propagated from inflamed texture and to be the consequence of a general disease of every part of the gland rather than of a new structure; furthermore, the spleen was also involved, thickly pervaded with bodies of various sizes resembling the structure of the diseased glands".

Hodgkin made no claim to priority and made no further study

of the condition. He seems to have been hesitant about writing at all, for he said: "Trust that I shall at least escape severe or general censure, even though a sentence or two should be produced from some existing work, couched in such concise but expressive language as to render needless the longer details with which I shall trespass on the time of my hearers". The account was largely unnoticed but Richard Bright (1789-1855) recognised it as the description of a new disease. In 1856 Samuel Wilks of Guy's (1824-1911) described, independently, "enlargement of the lymphatic glands combined with a peculiar disease of the spleen" and only learned later of Hodgkin's paper. General recognition did not result until Wilks wrote another paper in 1865 entitled "Cases of Enlargement of the Lymphatic Glands and Spleen (or Hodgkin's Disease)". "Although my own observations were at the time (1856) original, I had been forestalled by Dr Hodgkin who was the first, as far as I am aware, to call attention to this peculiar form of disease". The condition is now regarded as a malignant reticulosis.

Thomas Hodgkin's story is a rather sad one of failure and only posthumous recognition of some of his achievements. He was born at Tottenham on 6th January 1798 and educated at home and on the Continent. He began his medical training at Guy's Hospital and, after a year's extra study in Paris, he graduated M.D. Edinburgh in 1821. He learned stethoscopy from Laennec and was largely responsible for the introduction of the stethoscope to England. He was one of the first group of licentiates of the Royal College of Physicians of London to be selected by the Council for the Fellowship but declined the honour. (There were no Members at that time, 1825). In the newly-established museum at Guy's he became curator and worked on the classification of the specimens. He was lecturer in morbid anatomy and ran the first regular course on it in England. In the next 12 years he did all the work which made him eminent and gained for him the membership of scientific societies at home and abroad, including those of Boston and Philadelphia.

Hodgkin was a very humble man and somewhat lacking in worldly wisdom. He had a disregard for fees and the story is told of how he sat up all night with a wealthy patient who, on recovery, gave him a blank cheque. Hodgkin made it out for only £10. When the patient remonstrated Hodgkin naively said that he did not look as if he could afford more. Although never in robust health he had untiring energy and his mental vigour was present to the end of his life. Apart from Hodgkin's disease his name might have become eponymous for several other reasons, for he described aortic valvular insufficiency five years before Corrigan (1802-1880) and recorded the findings in acute appendicitis 60 years before Fitz's classic account of 1886 (Medical Classics 1938 2 459 Reprint).

Hodgkin suffered a great disappointment in 1837 and resigned from Guy's when he was passed over in favour of Dr Babbington for the position of assistant physician, a post which he greatly desired. His students and friends were greatly upset and charged the treasurer with having rejected Hodgkin because he was a Quaker of liberal activities who used the distinctive form of speech and dress of the Society of Friends. After this Hodgkin continued to practise in London but gradually forsook medicine and devoted himself to philanthropic work. He was in advance of his time in the reforms he advocated in medical education and practice. He stressed the value of necropsies and is said to have performed 250 in a year. He was an expert linguist and interested in dialects. In a paper read to the Philological Society he suggested that the Cockney dialect in which "v" is substituted for "w" was due to the speaker's partial deafness.

Hodgkin's activities in the Aborigines Protection Society and with oppressed people everywhere brought him the friendship of Sir Moses Montefiore Bt (1784-1885), an admirable example of how devotion to philanthropy brought together an orthodox Jew and steadfast Quaker. Hodgkin died at the age of 68 of "dysentery" when on a visit to Palestine with his friend on 4th April 1886. He had gone there on an errand of mercy to try to relieve the poverty and misery of the Jewish people in Jaffa. Sir Moses had an obelisk of Aberdeen granite erected at his grave "in commemoration of a friendship of more than 40 years". The epitaph was inscribed by his sorrowing widow. The graveyard, now disused, is behind the Tabeetha School of the Church of Scotland, at 21 Yeffet Street, Jaffa, Israel.

HORNER'S SYNDROME
Johann Friedrich Horner 1831-1886

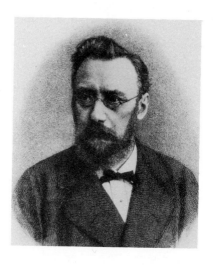

UNILATERAL constriction of the pupil, sinking-in of the eyeball, narrowing of the palpebral fissure, together with disturbance of flushing and sweating of the face and neck and blocking of the nose, constitute Horner's syndrome. It is caused by interference with the cervical sympathetic chain and its cerebral connections. Although others contributed to its discovery, Horner was the first to recognise its full significance as a lateralising rather than as a localising sign. The effect of stimulating the cervical sympathetic chain had been known for a century but Horner was unaware of this. In France the picture is referred to as the Claude Bernard-Horner syndrome and in Germany it is called Budge's phenomenon after the physiologist Johann Budge whose work to some extent anticipated that of Horner. Edward Sellick (1812-1838), a house surgeon at the Staffordshire Royal Infirmary, in discussing the case of a rapidly growing tumour of the neck, came very near to describing the features published by Horner 30 years later. He did not pursue the subject further, for he died from typhus a few days after his paper was published.

The following passage is taken from Horner's article, "Concerning a form of ptosis", in Klinische Monatsblätter Augenheilkunde 1869 7 193. The patient was a 40-year-old woman.

> *"Six weeks after the last pregnancy that occurred a year before I saw her, the patient noticed a gradual drooping of the right upper eyelid . . . the pupil of the right eye was found to be definitely smaller than that of the left, the eyeball was very slightly shrunken. . . . While the case was under observation there developed before our eyes gradually increasing redness and heat of the right half of the face although the left half remained pale and cold . . . The patient then told us for the first time that she had never perspired on the right side . . . I believe that in view of all these symptoms no-one will question my opinion that this gradually developing, but never complete, ptosis should be regarded as a paralysis of the superior palpebral muscle which is supplied by the sympathetic. I thus regard the phenomenon in the upper lid as part of a larger symptom complex".*

Johann Friedrich Horner was born in Zürich on 27th March 1831 and was the son of a physician. His mother, a highly cultivated woman, prided herself, like many Swiss, on her linguistic powers and taught her numerous offspring several languages. Johann studied the classics, natural history and mathematics in primary school in Zürich. After his military service he entered the university in 1849. Both his parents died while he was a student there. His interest in natural history soon led him to study medicine. He was a pupil of Carl Ludwig, the great experimental physiologist, who grounded him in the scientific method. Horner took his doctor's degree with the highest honours in 1854 for a thesis on curvature of the spine. He visited Munich and Vienna and became interested in ophthalmology. Von Jaeger, the eminent ophthalmologist, showed him the first volume of the newly-founded Archiv für Ophthalmologie of Albrecht von Graefe. A warm friendship sprang up between master and pupil which lasted until von

Graefe's death in 1870. In Paris, his next centre of study, he worked under Desmarres and published his first paper on constitutional disease detectable with the ophthalmoscope.

Horner made a great impression on his teachers and received tempting offers of posts in several places but after a year of travel he returned to his native land. He practised general medicine for some years and did not specialise in ophthalmology until 1861. In 1862 he was appointed professor of ophthalmology at Zürich and continued active in research and practice until his death on 20th December 1886. He wrote widely on ophthalmology and also left an uncompleted autobiography which was edited by the ophthalmologist, Edmund Landolt, in 1887.

HUNTINGTON'S CHOREA
George Huntington 1850-1916

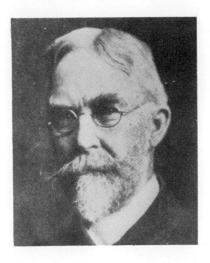

HUNTINGTON's name has become eponymous as a result of his only written medical communication, "On chorea", which he read before the Meigs and Mason Academy of Medicine in Middleport, Ohio, when he was 22. It was published in The Medical and Surgical Reporter, Philadelphia, 1872 26 317. His subject was chorea minor (Sydenham 1642-89) and he regarded the hereditary chorea he described as a particular form of Sydenham's chorea. After this he did not investigate chorea further and modestly refused to consider his description of major importance.

Hereditary chorea had probably existed throughout the ages though it has not been traced back further than the late 16th century. Between 1841 and 1885 it was described independently in America, Norway, England and Austria. Osler contributed a Festschrift to the Huntington number of Neurographs 1908 by William Browning in which he mentions reports of 1842 (C. O. Waters in Dunglison's Practice of Medicine) and 1863 (Irving W.

73

Lyon) and an endemic centre of hereditary chorea in Wyoming City, Pennsylvania (C. R. Gorman). An inherited form of chorea had been described also in Norway in 1859 by John Christian Lund. But it was Huntington who gave the first good account and called attention to the three characteristic features: its hereditary nature, the accompanying insanity and the fact that it appeared in middle life. It is now known to be transmitted by a rare autosomal Mendelian dominant gene.

The disease came to America in 1630 when the John Winthrop Puritan fleet with 700 persons anchored in Boston harbour. Among the passengers were five who were related from Bures, near Colchester, close to the Suffolk-Essex border. The men were Jeffers, Nick and Willis (fictitious names). Nick and Willis were brothers and the wives of Jeffers and Nick were sisters. Two sisters of the wives of Jeffers and Nick arrived soon afterwards.

Huntington's first encounter with the disease is described in his own words as follows:

"Over fifty years ago, in riding with my father on his rounds I saw my first case of "the disorder", which was the way the natives always referred to the dreaded disease. I recall it as vividly as though it had occurred but yesterday. It made a most enduring impression upon my boyish mind, an impression which was the very first impulse to my choosing chorea as my virgin contribution to medical lore. Driving with my father through a wooded road leading from East Hampton to Amagansett we suddenly came upon two women, mother and daughter, both tall, thin, almost cadaverous, both howling, twisting, grimacing. I stared in wonderment, almost in fear. What could it mean? My father paused to speak with them and we passed on. Then my Gamaliel-like instruction began; my medical instruction had its inception. From this point on my interest in the disease has never wholly ceased".

George Huntington was born in East Hampton, Long Island, on 9th April 1850, where his father, Abel Huntington, and grandfather, George Lee Huntington, were physicians and all familiar with hereditary chorea. His early medical training was from his father and then at the College of Physicians and Surgeons of Columbia University where he graduated at the age of 21. He practised for a time with his father and then moved to Palmyra, Ohio, but he spent most of his life in Dutchess County, New York. He was the archetype of the general practitioner or personal physician, a gentle nature-lover, highly regarded by his patients and an avid reader of medical journals. He was very fond of music and played the flute. He retired in 1915 and died the following year at the age of 66.

JACKSONIAN EPILEPSY
John Hughlings Jackson 1835-1911

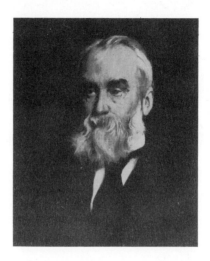

JACKSON defined epilepsy as "an occasional, sudden, excessive, rapid, local discharge of the gray matter". In the epileptic attack associated with his name the fit or convulsive movement is localised, and consciousness is only lost late, if at all. Jackson's more important contribution to neurology was his concept of a series of forces controlling movement" from the most voluntary to the most involuntary". He put forward his theory of levels in the central nervous system in 1875. On the more practical side he did much to promote the use of the ophthalmoscope. He was not a good lecturer, for he spoke mainly over the heads of his students.

John Hughlings Jackson was born at Providence Green, Green Hammerton, near Knaresborough, Yorkshire, on 4th April 1835. He was one of five children of Samuel Jackson, a farmer and small brewer. His mother, Sarah Hughlings, was of Welsh extraction. At the local school he gained a knowledge of French and always regretted that he did not learn German. On leaving school he was apprenticed to Mr Anderson at the York Dispensary and attended a small medical school in York where his lifelong friend, Johnathan Hutchinson (later Sir Johnathan Hutchinson, the famous surgeon), had been a student. He then proceeded to St Bartholomew's Hospital, London, where he obtained the qualifications usual in those days — Member of the Royal College of Surgeons and Licenciate of the Society of Apothecaries. In 1860 he became M.D. St Andrews. He spent the next three years in York as a house surgeon before deciding to return to London. At that time he thought of abandoning medicine for philosophy but Hutchinson dissuaded him. His decision to specialise in neurology is attributed to an attack of Bell's palsy. In 1862 Jackson became a member of the staff of the National Hospital for the Paralysed and Epileptic in Queen Square, London (see footnote p. 156), which had been founded two years earlier and where he worked for the next 45 years.

Jackson married his first cousin when aged 30, and she died 11 years later of cerebral thrombosis, associated ironically with Jacksonian epilepsy. Passionately fond of children, he had none of his own and, after his wife's death, he became rather eccentric. He always showed contempt for anything of the nature of red tape. Always restless and easily fatigued, he rarely sat a dinner out or saw a play to the last act. He relaxed by reading cheap novels but had no hobbies. He is said to have had the habit, when he bought a book, of tearing off the covers and then the book itself into half. He would stuff one half into each of his coat pockets and leave the shop assistant astonished. He was rarely seen at any public function and had no interest in music or sport. Food did not interest him and he always hurried through his meals. He did not smoke. He was an agnostic and an absolute disbeliever in personal immortality. He died of pneumonia at 3 Manchester Square, London, on 11th November 1911 when aged 76. Jackson's fame has grown continuously since his death and his neurological doctrines have become firmly established.

KOPLIK'S SPOTS
Henry Koplik 1858-1927

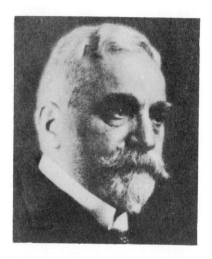

KOPLIK described his spots in the Archives of Pediatrics (New York) 1896 13 918 in an article entitled "The diagnosis of the invasion of measles from a study of the exanthem as it appears on the buccal mucous membrane". But the profession did not seem to recognise their importance and further articles were needed. They were characteristic of Koplik's perseverance and forcible will in pressing for their recognition. Now the spots are well known to all. Describing the inside of the lips in the 24 to 48 hours before the rash of measles appears, Koplik said:

"On the buccal mucous membrane and the inside of the lips we invariably see a distinct eruption. It consists of small irregular spots of bright red colour. In the centre of each spot is noted in strong daylight a minute bluish-white speck . . . These red spots . . . are absolutely pathognomonic of measles".

It would have been remarkable if these spots had remained unreported until Koplik's time and we find that in 1774 John Quier in Jamaica described "aphthous specks about the gums which are always visible several days before the eruption". (The life and scientific works of Dr John Quier, practitioner of physic and surgery, Jamaica, 1738-1822. H. Goerke. West Indian Medical Journal 1956 5 23). Others who described them were Richard Hazeltine, a general practitioner in Maine, in 1802; Flindt, a Danish physician, in 1885, and Carl Gerhardt in 1881. Filatov, the father of paediatrics in Russia, described the spots in 1885 and emphasised the desquamative eruption, whereas Koplik laid stress on the bluish-white spots. Russian pre-revolutionary literature refers to Koplik's spots but now in the U.S.S.R. they are known as Filatov's sign. Osler and Henoch also mention them but no author gave as precise a description as Koplik did or insisted that they were the prodromal sign of measles and that they occurred in no other disease. The eponym rightly belongs to him for pressing their importance in the diagnosis of measles in the pre-eruptive stage.

Henry Koplik was born in New York City on 2nd October 1858. Little is known of his early life. He received his M.D. from the College of Physicians and Surgeons of Columbia University in 1881. He then spent several years studying in Berlin, Vienna and Prague. His first appointment was to the Good Samaritan Dispensary where he started a "baby health station" at which milk was supplied for infants at six bottles for eight cents (200 were given free). He told the story of the foundation of this clinic in an article, "The history of the first milk depots or Gouttes de Lait with consultations in America" (Journal of the American Medical Association 1914 50 1574). Koplik was attending paediatrician at Mount Sinai Hospital for 25 years where he was foremost in urging the use of the laboratory in clinical medicine. He was also consulting physician to the Jewish Maternity Hospital and the Hebrew Orphan Asylum. His book, "The Diseases of Infancy and Childhood", appeared in 1902 and went to four editions. Its words showed a certain human sympathy so often lacking in scientific literature.

Koplik was a big handsome man with a white van Dyke beard, a moustache, and bushy eyebrows overhanging his flashing dark eyes. He had a sparkling wit and an inexhaustible fund of anecdotes. His ward rounds were conducted with military precision and inspired awe in those around him. In later life he made many trips abroad and often introduced into his wards innovations he saw and approved of. He died of coronary thrombosis in New York on 30th April 1927, aged 69.

KORSAKOV'S PSYCHOSIS
Sergei Sergeivich Korsakov 1854-1900

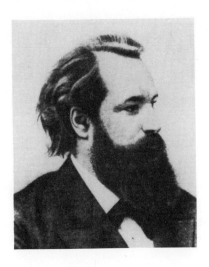

THE amnestic confabulatory syndrome which he called
"cerebropathia psychica toxaemica" was described by Korsakov
in a thesis which in 1887 gained him the degree of M.D. He
published a description of the syndrome in a Russian journal,
Vestnik Psychiatrie, under the title "Disturbances in the psychic
sphere occurring in alcoholic paralysis and their relation to the
psychic disturbances in multiple neuritis of non-alcoholic
origin". A second article, entitled "A peculiar form of psychic
disturbance associated with peripheral neuritis", was published
in a leading German journal (Allgemeine Zeitschrift für
Psychiatrie 1889-90 46 475) and this found a wider circle of readers.

There had been earlier accounts of the condition. Dr James
Jackson (1777-1868), of Boston, the first physician to the
Massachusetts General Hospital, had given an account of
alcoholic neuritis in 1822 but made only brief mention of the
mental symptoms. A fuller account, with a masterly description of

81

the mental symptoms, was published by the great Guy's clinician, Sir Samuel Wilks (1824-1911), in the Medical Times and Gazette (1868 2 467) under the title "Alcoholic paraplegia". Wilks wrote: "Most of my examples were those of women or, as I say, 'ladies', as the patients were usually publicans' wives and their husbands were landlords". In 1868 Wilks considered that the cord and membrances were involved but said in his reminiscences (1911) that later investigations had shown that the disease was a chronic neuritis.

The characteristic mental symptoms to which Korsakov drew attention were loss of memory for recent events ("they literally forget everything immediately") and pseudo-reminiscences. Although this picture can occur in other disorders, the eponymous term is used nowadays only when the condition is associated with alcoholic peripheral neuritis.

Sergei Sergeivich Korsakov was born on the Gus estate in Vladimir province, in Russia, on 22nd January 1854. He studied medicine in Moscow, graduating in 1875. After working at the Preobrazhenski mental hospital and as assistant to A. J. Kozhevnikov, professor of neurology and psychiatry, he was himself appointed "extraordinary professor" in 1892. He succeeded to the full professorship in 1889 and held the chair until his death. He published a textbook of psychiatry (in Russian) in 1893 and many articles on neurology, psychiatry and medical jurisprudence.

Korsakov was greatly respected for his humanitarianism. Even when a boy of 11, he wrote: "Help others. When the occasion presents itself to do good deeds, do them. Withdraw from evil". He remained true to this principle throughout his life. Even apart from the syndrome which bears his name, Korsakov deserves a place in medical history as the first great psychiatrist of Russia. In many ways he was in advance of his time, for he advocated the "no restraint" principle and freed his patients from straitjackets. He was chairman of the Society for Aid to Needy Students and in 1890 was largely responsible for the founding of the Moscow Society of Neuropathologists and Psychiatrists. Another project of wider scope was the foundation of the Russian Association of

Psychiatrists and Neurologists and it is sad to record that Korsakov died on 1st May 1900, at the early age of 46, just before this Association came into being.

DOWN'S SYNDROME
John Langdon Haydon Langdon-Down
1828-1896

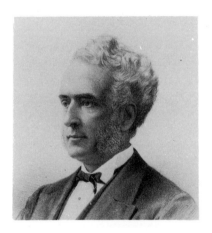

Down's syndrome is now replacing the term, mongolism — a term which has perpetuated the mistaken idea that this type of mental subnormality is found only in races with some mongolian ancestry. This is clearly untrue, for mongolism is found in all races, including those of pure Negro stock.

Down's article on "Observations on an ethnic classification of idiots", published in 1866, gave the first comprehensive description of mongolism. In it, he maintained that certain classes of mental defective had similar peculiarities which seemed to place them within specific ethnological families. His theory was further elaborated by Francis Crookshank (1873-1933) in his book, "The Mongol in our Midst". In 1959, the finding of a small extra chromosome in the cells of three mongol patients resulted in mongolism being recognised as one of the disorders associated with chromosome anomalies. In view of this, and out of consideration for the Mongol race, modern practice uses the more appropriate name, "Down's syndrome".

Down was born on 18th November 1828 at Torpoint, Cornwall, which is opposite Plymouth. His father was of Irish descent and his mother a member of a well-known family, the Langdons of Devon. His early education was at a dames' school and then, at the age of 11, he attended the Devonport Classical and Mathematical School where he was a bright pupil and regularly at the top of his form. After two years he left school to help in his father's apothecary's business. At 18, he went to London and after a brief period with a surgeon in Whitechapel he entered the laboratory of the Pharmaceutical Society. His intention was to become a scientist but his progress was halted by a call back to the family business and a period of ill-health.

After his father died in 1848, Down decided to study medicine having been persuaded that science was too precarious a career. On 1st October 1853, at the age of 25, he became a medical student at The London Hospital. In 1856 he obtained the Licence of the Society of Apothecaries and Membership of the Royal College of Surgeons — the usual qualifications in those days. In 1858, after holding several posts at The London Hospital, including those of medical tutor, resident accoucheur and lecturer in comparative anatomy, he became medical superintendent at Earlswood Asylum for Idiots, at Redhill, Surrey. In the same year he obtained the degree of M.B. and a gold medal in physiology. The next year he became M.D. and M.R.C.P. and was appointed assistant physician to The London Hospital. He was elected F.R.C.P. in 1868 in which year, after spending ten years at Earlswood, he left to take up private practice in London, at 81 Harley Street, and to start with his wife a home at Teddington, Middlesex, for the training of feeble-minded children. This building, which had been known as the White House, was renamed Normansfield in memory of an intimate friend and helper, Norman Wilkinson. The institution grew rapidly and eventually had 200 patients. After Down's death, Normansfield was administered by his two sons, and later by his grandson, so that for over 100 years its physician-superintendent was a member of Down's family. In 1952 the hospital was taken over by the National Health Service.

Down is described as a large man with a handsome face. He had great charm and was one of Nature's gentlemen. His unvarying gentleness gave him an extraordinary influence over his unfortunate patients. Whilst he lived up to the highest principles, he was no ascetic and was always a most genial host. Down's name might have well become eponymous for his other work, for, in his "Mental Affections of Childhood and Youth", he gave a detailed account of dystrophia adiposo-genitalis 40 years before Frölich described it. In many ways Down was in advance of his time. He advocated higher education for women and denied that this would make them more liable to produce feeble-minded children.

McARDLE'S DISEASE
Brian McArdle born 1911

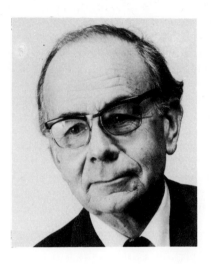

BRIAN MCARDLE became interested in muscle diseases soon after taking up a clinical research post in Cambridge in 1936. He was able to study two cases of periodic paralysis and this aroused an interest both in potassium metabolism and in the rapidly expanding field of muscle biochemistry. He had intended to continue this work at the National Hospital for Nervous Diseases, Queen Square, London, but World War II interrupted these studies. He joined a team at the "National" investigating motion sickness, the treatment of sea sickness and the effects of working in severe heat. He had been trained at Guy's Hospital and returned there in 1947 as a member of the Medical Research Council's Clinical Research Unit. He resumed his interest in the carbohydrate metabolism of muscle disease and developed techniques for its investigation. The condition with which McArdle's name is associated is phosphorylase deficiency of muscle — type V of the glycogenoses — a rare, non-progressive benign disorder of glycogen storage unaffected by treatment.

The patient, "Georgie", with this condition had been spotted by the late Dr A. C. Hampson as an instance of probable metabolic disorder of muscle. His chief complaint was of pain and stiffness on exercise, even that of chewing. "Georgie" was 30 but the symptoms had been present since childhood. There were no abnormalities on routine examination, but ischaemic exercise of the forearm rapidly induced a painful shortening of the flexor muscles which, since they were shown to be electro-myographically silent, originated in the fibres themselves. Blood flow on exercise was considerably greater than normal. Investigation showed that the muscles did not produce any lactic acid even during ischaemic exercise. McArdle concluded from this latter finding, and from the demonstration of contractures provoked by exercise, that the condition was "a myopathy due to a defect in muscle glycogen breakdown" (the title of his paper in Clinical Science 1951 10 13). Eight years later it was shown that phosphorylase was absent from the muscles of patients with this disorder. Many years after this, McArdle studied in another case the cause of the stiffness and contracture that can be a striking feature during, and following, severe or ischaemic exercise. McArdle's abiding interest has been in the metabolic disorders of muscle, and especially in the familial periodic paralyses, but for some years he also worked on biochemical aspects of peripheral neuropathies and of multiple sclerosis.

Brian McArdle* was born in London on 9th April 1911 and educated at Wimbledon College and Guy's Hospital Medical School. He qualified in 1933 and obtained his M.D. and M.R.C.P. in 1936. He was elected F.R.C.P. in 1966. He now works in the Department of Chemical Pathology at Guy's Hospital on the external scientific staff of the Medical Research Council.

---

*Not to be confused with Michael John Francis McArdle, neurologist to Guy's Hospital and the National Hospital, Queen Square, London.

MACEWEN'S OSTEOTOMY
MACEWEN'S SUPRAMEATAL
TRIANGLE
Sir William Macewen 1848-1924

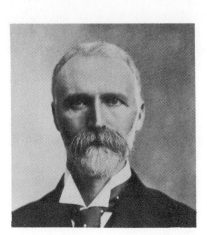

THIS "austere and majestic giant" was one of the great figures in the surgical world in the second half of the 19th century. He was born on 22nd June 1848 near Rothesay, on the Isle of Bute, in the Firth of Clyde, the youngest in a family of 12. His father was a master mariner. He attended the Rothesay Academy until he was 12 when his parents moved to Glasgow. An intelligent boy, but indifferent to books and in no way precocious, he was more at home in the gymnasium than in the classroom. His favourite pastime was sailing and his hobby biology, but he had no interest in the usual sports. At Glasgow University he matriculated at 17. In his medical course he was taught by several distinguished men, including Lord Lister whom he revered. As a student he experimented with heat sterilisation at the time when antiseptic surgery was giving place to aseptic techniques. He graduated M.B., C.M. in 1869 and M.D. in 1872. His first post, after house appointments, was as medical superintendent of the Glasgow

Fever Hospital at Belvidere and it was there that he developed the technique of laryngeal intubation for diptheria.

As was the custom, he spent a period in general practice and gave this up on becoming a dispensary surgeon. In 1874 he was appointed to the junior staff of the Glasgow Royal Infirmary and two years later was surgeon-in-charge of wards. In those days the appointment was for a fixed term of 15 years and this would have brought Macewen's retirement at the age of 48. In recognition of his outstanding service the Board of Management reappointed him for a second term. In 1892 he moved to the Western Infirmary to be regius professor of surgery in the University of Glasgow. At one stage he had been invited to the chair of surgery at Johns Hopkins Medical School, Baltimore, but the project was dropped and he continued in Glasgow until his death at the age of 75.

Macewen was a man of impressive and handsome appearance, six feet two inches tall, with clear blue eyes and the look of a Viking, so that he was sometimes mistaken for a soldier. He had immense energy, was highly articulate and of impeccable integrity. Proudly conscious of his own pre-eminence, he had few intimates. As a teacher he was extremely emphatic and it is said that his students learned two sets of surgical dogma to be used at the Royal or the Western Infirmary as the circumstances demanded. He did not have the humility of Lister and seems to have felt that God had delegated to him the practice of surgery of which he could be regarded as a Cecil Rhodes, a Wellington or a Nelson. That he was in many ways an autocrat cannot be denied, but since his death stories of his great kindness to patients show that there was another aspect to his character. Sir D'Arcy Power called him "the unfair surgeon" because he was exhaustive in his work and left little for aftercomers to improve or amend. David Ligat, a surgeon at St Leonard's-on-Sea, recorded that he (David Ligat) once asked his chief, Sir Alfred Pearce Gould, who he thought was the greatest surgeon of the century. Without hesitation the reply was: Kocher or Macewen, and I think Macewen just has it"

Macewen extended many fields of surgery, for, as well as developing the aseptic method and laryngeal intubation, he introduced bone-grafting and osteotomy, and operated successfully for brain abscess and fracture of the patella. He perfected the surgical approach to the middle ear and in 1893 described the supra-meatal fossa in a book "Pyogenic diseases of the brain and Spinal Cord", Glasgow Maclehose) as follows:

"Roughly speaking, if the orifice of the external osseous meatus be bisected horizontally, the upper half would be on the level of the mastoid antrum. If this segment be again bisected vertically its posterior half would again correspond to the junction of the antrum and the middle ear and immediately behind this lies the suprameatal fossa".

The operation of femoral osteotomy for knock knee was described in a remarkable book on osteotomy in which Macewen recorded that he operated on 557 limbs in 330 patients with only three deaths. Many would regard him as virtually the creator of the specialities of cerebral, thoracic and orthopaedic surgery. In no sense a team worker, he left behind no Macewen school of surgery. He preferred to work out his problems by himself and once, when asked to take charge of a project to establish a hospital for limbless ex-servicemen, replied: "I'll take it up on one condition — that you do not ask other surgeons to co-operate; I am not a co-operator".

Macewen married Mary Watson Allan and they had three sons and three daughters. He died on 22nd March 1924 of pneumonia.

SCHISTOSOMA MANSONI
Sir Patrick Manson 1844-1922

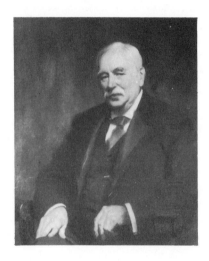

MANSON'S interest in worms began in boyhood and there is a prophetic story that when he shot a cat on his father's farm he was found examining a tape worm inside it. The story of how his name became eponymous begins with the prevalent haematuria of Egypt, about the cause of which nothing was known until Theodor Bilharz, a young German comparative anatomist, working in Egypt, found the causal parasite in 1851. He called it *Distomum haematobium*. T. S. Cobbold (1828-1888), the British authority on parasites, pointed out that it was not a *distomum* and proposed the name, Bilharzia, in honour of its discoverer. Three months earlier the name, *Schistosoma*, had been suggested by David Weinland. *Bilharzia haematobium* was accepted as the cause of bilharzia for half-a-century and British soldiers even had a slang equivalent, "Bill Harris". Those who later tightened up the rules of zoological nomenclature allowed the three months priority to stand and the name *Schistosoma haematobium* was adopted. In 1902 Manson found schistosome eggs with lateral spines in the faeces of a patient from Antigua. He knew that eggs in the urine had terminal spines and found it difficult to believe that a worm could lay eggs of different structure in different organs and suggested that there was more than one species of parasite. This proved to be the case and, 65 years after the discovery of Bilharz, the parasites were distinguished and *Schistosoma mansoni* was established as the parasite causing intestinal schistosomiasis.

Patrick Manson was born on 3rd December 1844 at Cromlett Hill, Old Meldrum, Aberdeenshire, the second son of John Manson, a laird of Fingask and manager of the local bank. The family moved to Aberdeen where Patrick attended the West End Academy. His first intention was to become an engineer, but the heavy work and weakness of his right arm forced him to give up his apprenticeship. He entered Aberdeen University in 1860 and passed the final examination at the age of 20, spending the time, until he was old enough to take the degrees of M.B., C.M., in visiting hospitals and museums in London. In 1865 he became M.D. with a thesis on the internal carotid artery, written when he was medical officer to the Durham Lunatic Asylum. Immediately afterwards he took a post in the Far East as medical officer to the Chinese Imperial Maritime Customs at Takao, Formosa.

After eight years in Formosa, political unrest caused him to leave and he transferred to Amoy on the Chinese mainland. Here he did similar work for 13 years but also had charge of a hospital for European seaman and a missionary hospital. He started teaching at the new Alice Memorial Hospital, the precursor of the medical school of Hong Kong. It was customary in those days for Chinese physicians to examine their patients in the street and Manson imitated them by seeing his patients in a front room with a large window. He was accepted by the Chinese and practised in Hong Kong for six years from December 1883, becoming a great personality in the district. The confidence of the local population was gained by his successful removal of a large elephantoid tumour from a man who had failed in attempted suicide and thought that, as he could not kill himself, Manson might as well do it.

Manson took home leave very infrequently and, when he did, he used to spend it working in the British Museum, sitting, it is said, on the opposite side of a table at which Karl Marx was writing "Das Kapital".

Manson's observations on filariasis played an important part in making the first great discovery in tropical medicine, namely that human diseases could be spread by winged insects. Embryos of filaria worms had been found in the blood and urine by Timothy Lewis in 1870-72. Manson found the adult worm, *Filaria bancrofti*, in the scrotum of a patient in 1887, but, until he worked on the problem, the life history of the worm was only partly known. A puzzling feature of filariasis was the presence of embryos in the blood at night but not during the day. This suggested to Manson that the habits of filariae were adapted to those of the mosquito which he guessed was carrying them. His theory was proved correct when he persuaded his servant, Buito, who had filariae in his blood, to sleep in a mosquito cage. He found that over the next few days filariae had migrated from the insects' stomachs to the muscles. To use his own words, he had "stumbled upon an important fact with a distinct bearing on human pathology". But he did not complete the story correctly and thought the mosquito died after ovipositing and so set free embryos to infect drinking water. It was not until 1889 that the younger Bancroft showed that filariae actively developed in certain types of mosquito and were transferred by the act of feeding on blood.

Manson's interest in worms was lifelong and, even when he settled in London, he kept his knowledge of them up-to-date. He played a part in the discovery of the lung fluke, *Paragonimus westermani*, and a parasitic worm of dogs and cats, *Diphyllobothrium mansoni*.

Manson's work on malaria did not bring him any entitlement to eponymity but it played a big part in showing the mode of transmission of the disease and so helped in its eradication from large areas of the world. Having established that insects could be vectors of disease, he advanced the hypothesis that the malaria parasite (discovered by Laveran in 1880) was carried by mosquitoes. He published this in the British Medical Journal 1894 2 1306. In this year Manson met Ronald Ross (1845-1922), who had worked on the life cycle of the malaria parasite, and this stimulated him to further work which showed the pigmented cystic stage of the parasite in 1897 and, in 1898, its presence in the salivary glands of the mosquito. The final link in the chain was established by Manson who, in 1900, obtained from Italy some mosquitoes which had fed on a malarial patient. His son, Thorburn, allowed himself to be bitten by them and two weeks later had undoubted malaria. Ross was awarded the Nobel Prize in 1902 and in his Nobel lecture acknowledged his indebtedness to Manson.

Manson had planned to retire to Scotland in 1890, at the early age of 46, but his role as a country gentleman at Kildrummy, on Donside, lasted for less than a year. The investments he had made did not prosper and so he resumed practice, this time at 21 Queen Anne Street, London. At the end of his first year in practice he became M.R.C.P. by examination. He gave lectures on tropical medicine at St George's, Charing Cross and the Royal Free Hospitals. At this time there was no special place for the study of tropical diseases and Manson's greatest work, and the one which earned him the title of "The Father of Tropical Medicine", was the founding of the London School of Tropical Medicine.

Manson spent the year 1875 on holiday in England and in December of that year married Henrietta Isabella Thorburn. He was a big handsome man, fond of outdoor life, and looked more like a country squire than a man immersed in medical problems. Often laid low by gout, he worked almost to the end of his life, being wheeled from bed to bed on his later ward rounds. The last post he held was that of medical adviser to the Colonial Office and when he retired from it he settled at The Sheiling, on Lough Mask, Co. Galway, Ireland, where he died on 9th April 1922.

MECKEL'S DIVERTICULUM
Johann Friedrich Meckel the younger
1781-1833

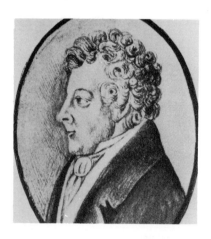

In the latter half of the 18th century and the first half of the 19th century there existed in Germany what can be called a Meckel scientific dynasty. Between 1748 and 1856 there were only a few years when the Meckels were not directing the studies of normal and pathological anatomy in Germany. The name of only one of them has remained eponymous and that from his description of what is usually called Meckel's diverticulum — an unobliterated residuum of the vitello-intestinal duct which is found at the lower end of the ileum in about two per cent of people. When inflamed or bleeding (from ulcerated ectopic gastric mucosa) it is a well-known pitfall for the surgeon. Others had noted it earlier but Meckel detailed its origin.

Johann Friedrich Meckel the younger bore the same forenames as his grandfather (1714-1774) who was teacher of anatomy, surgery, botany and obstetrics in Berlin and who described the spheno-palatine (Meckel's) ganglion. His father, Philip Friedrich Meckel (1756-1803), was professor of anatomy and surgery at Halle.

Johann Friedrich the younger was born in Halle on 13th October 1781 and went to school there until 1795. His father made him assist in preparing specimens for his anatomical collection but at that stage Johann was not inclined to follow a medical career. He enrolled as a medical student at Halle after a trip to St Petersburg with his father.

He graduated in 1802 with a thesis on congenital abnormalities of the heart and was soon working in the museums of Paris and Vienna. In 1806 he went to Italy to make some marine investigations but his stay was cut short when Napoleon invaded Prussia. Meckel is said to have crossed the Alps on foot in his haste to get back to Halle and his widowed step-mother. He found that Napoleon had made his headquarters in the family home and had disbanded the university. He continued his work nevertheless and when the university reopened in 1808 he succeeded to the chair of anatomy, pathological anatomy, surgery and obstetrics vacated by his father.

Meckel married in 1809 Friederike von Kleist, the daughter of the commandant of Halle. There were no children. Meckel was handsome with light blue eyes, blonde curly hair and expressive features. His witty and acute observations enlivened his conversation and lectures. In later life he showed paranoid symptoms and was involved in violent quarrels with his colleagues. In spite of the many honours which were showered on him he had a constant unsatisfied gnawing hunger for recognition as a scientist. Through his impulsive, domineering and irritable nature he subjected himself and those around him to great wear and tear. In spite of this he had charming and generous characteristics as well. From the age of about 50 he gradually withdrew from the world and found some degree of peace at Giebichenstein, on the Saale valley, where he died on 31st October 1833, aged 52.

Although Meckel is remembered today solely for the anatomical anomaly he described, he explored human anatomy in depth and greatly increased our knowledge. His conclusions anticipated

Darwin, for he said that the body developed according to laws which were valid for the whole animal kingdom and passed through stages of life which preceded it.

MENIÈRE'S DISEASE
Prosper Menière 1799-1862

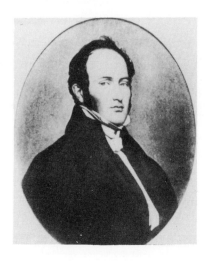

MENIÈRE'S paper, "On a particular kind of hearing loss resulting from a lesion of the inner ear", was read to the Imperial Academy of Medicine in Paris on 6th January 1861. There was no discussion. The title was improved on publication in the Gazette Médicale de Paris 1861 16 597 to "A report on lesions of the inner ear giving rise to symptoms of cerebral congestion of apoplectic type". Menière described "a young lady who, having travelled at night on the outside seat of a diligence while menstruating, caught a cold and suffered complete and sudden deafness". But the main symptom was "a continual vertigo; the slightest effort of moving produced vomiting". She died five days later. Of the post-mortem examination Menière wrote: "The only lesion I found was that the semi-circular canals were filled with a plastic (plastique) red matter". It is now thought probable that the girl had leukaemia, a rare background for Menière's symptom complex of deafness, tinnitus and vertigo. Menière's findings made him conclude that "the material lesion resides in the semi-circular canals" and thus he separated his clinical syndrome from the rag-bag of "apoplectiform cerebral congestion". All this occurred in the last year of Menière's life. The eponym has served us well for over 100 years and is likely to continue, for it has no hypothetical implications of other terms such as labyrinthine hydrops.

Prosper Menière was born at Angers on the Maine in France on 18th June 1799, the third of four children of a prosperous merchant. At the Lyçee he received an excellent education in the classics and the humanities. He was interested in botany and later became a member of the Linnean Society and a connoisseur of orchids. At the University of Angers he was an excellent student and won many prizes and medals. He completed his medical studies in Paris and became extern in 1822 and intern in 1823. He received his doctorate in 1828 and became clinical aide to Dupuytren at the Hôtel-Dieu where he had a strenuous and exciting time during "les troubles de Juillet" (1830). When Charles X abdicated and Louis Phillip ascended the throne Menière made the acquaintance of famous men in all walks of life — Victor Hugo, Ampère and Balzac — and became *persona grata* in many of the most select salons of Paris.

In 1832 Menière was involved as a physician in a political scene. When Charles X of France departed for England his daughter-in-law, the Duchess de Berri, widow of the murdered son of Charles X, followed him. The Duchess in due course returned to France to try to secure the throne for her 11-year-old son but she was betrayed and imprisoned in the Chateau de Blaye. She was guarded by General Bugeand and Menière was given the job of being her personal physician. A deep friendship arose between them. Menière found the Duchess to be pregnant and had to report the fact to the government. In due course a daughter was born. When her secret marriage to an Italian nobleman became known the Duchess lost all support for her plans and she returned to her husband in Sicily. Menière then returned in stages to Paris.

After this episode Menière was made chef de clinique to Chomel, a noted physician. For his part in organising assistance in an outbreak of cholera he was made a Chevalier of the Legion of

Honour. Despite his reputation and eminence he never achieved membership of the Académie de Medicine, although he was professionally eligible there were always candidates with better and nepotic claims.

In 1838 Menière became physician-in-chief to the Imperial Institute for Deaf Mutes and from that date his main interest was in diseases of the ear. A little known fact is that he made the crucial observation that improvement in hearing could follow mobilisation of the stapes. Menière was a prolific writer and his son said of him: "Il mettrait la plume volontiers à la main". He contributed weekly articles on matters of interest to the Gazette Médicale. In one of these, "Encore un mot sur la pellagre", he pointed out that spoiled maize and sunlight were not enough to explain all the facts. In "Etudes médicales sur les poetes latins" he combined his medical and literary interests.

Menière died very quickly of influenzal pneumonia on 7th February 1862 having been busy writing on the previous day. He had married Mlle Bequerel, a member of the distinguished family of scientists, in 1838 and their son, Emile Antoine Ménière,* became a noted otologist.

---

*Prosper wrote his name Menière but his son wrote Ménière.

DE MORGAN'S SPOTS
Campbell Greig de Morgan 1811-1876

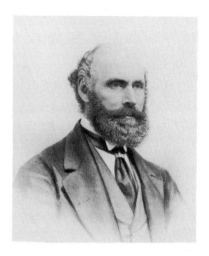

SMALL red spots are often found on the skin, especially of the chest and abdomen, of many elderly patients. These "de Morgan spots" were described by Campbell de Morgan, surgeon to the Middlesex Hospital, in The Lancet 1871 2 41. The article was one of a series on The Origin of Cancer which de Morgan republished as a book with the same title in 1872. De Morgan wrote:

"There is another circumstance in connexion with the recurrence of cancer after operation which to my mind is very significant. I have noticed, and it has been verified by the observation of many others, that, concurrently with or following on the development of cancer, small outgrowths of warty or vascular or dermoid structure are frequent. These cherry angiomas or ruby spots are well circumscribed, discrete, roughly circular lesions found mainly on the trunk and only rarely on hairy parts. They are composed of an

overgrowth of dilated vessels which show no pulsation and only slight blanching on pressure".

De Morgan regarded the spots as almost pathognomonic of cancer but, although his opinion at first had considerable support, they are no longer held to have the significance he attached to them. Sir John Bland-Sutton made careful observations on them for 25 years and found they were as common in the non-cancerous as in the cancerous ("Tumours, Innocent and Malignant" 7th edition 1922, 129). More recent studies by W. B. Bean (Transactions of the Association of American Physicians 1953 66 240) of over 1,000 patients have shown that they are not the hallmark of cancer. An outbreak of these spots in Lancashire in 1968 suggested an ingested factor, possibly in food, as the cause (Seville R. H. et al British Medical Journal 1970 1 408).

Campbell de Morgan was born at Clovelly, near Bideford, Devon, in 1811, the youngest of three sons of Colonel de Morgan, of the Indian Army. His elder brother was Augustus, the famous mathematician who wrote "A Budget of Paradoxes". Colonel de Morgan died when his sons were very young and they owed more than most children to the care and training they received from their mother. Campbell was educated at University College and the Middlesex Hospital qualifying M.R.C.S. in 1835. In 1842 he was appointed assistant surgeon to the Middlesex Hospital and the following year became one of the 300 original Fellows of the newly-chartered Royal College of Surgeons of England. He became full surgeon in 1847.

In collaboration with Mr (afterwards Sir) John Tomes he contributed to the Philosophical Transactions of 1852, a valuable paper on the structure and development of bone which led to his election as a Fellow of the Royal Society in 1861. For 34 years he studied the problem of cancer in a special ward set up in the Middlesex Hospital by Sir Samuel Whitbread in 1792. But he was no specialist as is shown by the fact that he lectured successively on forensic medicine, anatomy, physiology and surgery and took charge of the ophthalmic department of the hospital after its inception in 1843. Having been associated with the Middlesex Hospital Medical School since its foundation in 1835 he came to occupy a position of exceptional authority and exerted a great influence on the students. He was a man of strong religious feelings and every act of his life was regulated by his own rigid laws of what was right; this made him some enemies. He was very strict and punctual in all his duties and held himself to a straight and narrow path. He was strong in condemning greed for fees and showed a seeming indifference to worldly success. His last act of kindness to a dying man corresponded to the tenor of his life, for on Thursday 6th April 1876 he sat up all night with his old friend, Lough, an artist, who died next day. He returned home in the cold early morning and the following day had a rigor, the start of an illness from which he died on 12th April.

OSLER'S NODES
Sir William Osler Bt 1849-1919

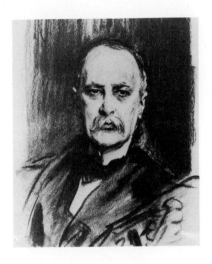

OSLER's name is most often remembered when we speak of Osler's nodes, one of the embolic phenomena of subacute bacterial endocarditis. They were first mentioned by Osler in an article on "The chronic intermittent fever of endocarditis" (Practitioner 1893 50 181) in which he says his attention was called to them by Dr Mullin (or Mullen), of Hamilton, Ontario. The patient was a spinster of 28 with mitral disease in whom "small spots appeared on the hands and feet, also on arms, legs and face, that looked like 'hives' ". In his classic paper in The Quarterly Journal of Medicine (1908-09 2 220) on Chronic Infectious Endocarditis, Osler described the "ephemeral spots of a painful nodular erythema", chiefly in the skin of the hands and feet, the "nodosites cutanees éphémères" of the French. Osler again records his indebtedness to Dr Mullen and quotes the latter's original description:

> "*The spots came out at intervals as small swollen areas, some the size of a pea, others a centimetre and a half in diameter,*

raised, red, with a whitish point in the centre. I have known them to pass away in a few hours, but more commonly they last for a day or even longer. The commonest situation is near the tip of the finger, which may be slightly swollen".

Osler adds: "They are not beneath but in the skin and they are not unlike an ordinary wheal of urticaria . . . I have never seen them haemorrhagic, but always erythematous, sometimes of a very vivid pink hue, with a slightly opaque centre".

Other conditions in which Osler's name is part of their eponym are Hereditary Haemorrhagic Telangiectasia (Rendu-Osler-Weber disease)* and Polycythaemia Vera (Osler-Vaquez disease)**. Osler entered the veterinary field with a paper on "Verminous Bronchitis in Dogs with a description of a new parasite" (The Veterinarian, London, 1877 1 387). Osler named the worm responsible *Strongylus canis bronchialis* but he mistook its generic identity and it was subsequently renamed *Filaria Osleri* by Cobbold in 1879.

William Osler, a Canadian of Celtic stock, was born at Bond Head, Ontario, on 12th July 1849, the sixth son and eighth child in a family of nine. His father, The Rev. Featherstone Lake Osler, had emigrated from Falmouth to do mission work in Canada. William at first intended to take holy orders but his love of natural history soon showed that his true vocation lay elsewhere. His medical training began at Toronto in 1868 and continued at McGill University, Montreal, where he graduated in 1872. He then made a long tour of European medical centres with Harvey Cushing and Thomas McCrae. It included 15 months in the physiological laboratory of University College, London, under Burdon Sanderson whom he was destined to follow as Regius Professor of Medicine at Oxford 34 years later. Here he was the first man to see the globoid bodies now known as platelets circulating in the blood. On a visit to London in 1878 he became M.R.C.P.

---

*Henri Jules Louis Rendu 1844-1962 French physician.

Frederick Parkes Weber 1863-1962 Physician to the German Hospital, London.

**Louis Henri Vaquez 1860-1936 French physician.

Osler's life was remarkable in that he became professor of medicine successively at four centres — Montreal 1874 (at the age of 25), Philadelphia 1884, Baltimore 1889 and Oxford 1904. It has been given to very few medical men to be invited to important positions in different countries in this way. In all of them he left the stamp of his powerful personality. His period at Baltimore was perhaps his most productive, for there he published his *magnum opus*, "The Principles and Practice of Medicine", in 1892. It ran to a 16th edition in 1947 and was translated into French, German, Spanish and Chinese. By 1905, 100,000 copies had been sold. William Morris, later Lord Nuffield, a great friend of Osler, declared that he would never think it worth consulting any doctor who did not have Osler's book clearly in use in his consulting room. For a long time he had wished to make his home in Britain and after the strain of his work in Baltimore he welcomed his translation in 1905 to the calm and cultured atmosphere of Oxford. Here he remained very active at the Radcliffe Infirmary and in University circles. At his home, The Open House, his hospitality was boundless.

Osler had little faith in drugs, and treatment was largely ineffective in his time. A favourite prescription of his was: "Time in divided doses". There are many tales about Osler. He used to remind his class of the advice of Oliver Wendell Holmes: "Not to take authority when he could take facts, not to guess when he could not know and not to think that a man must take physic because he is sick". A story which illustrates his interest in pathology is of an old man who begged alms. Osler gave him a coin and said "There is only one thing of value about you and that is your hob-nailed liver". Then he handed him his overcoat and added: "You may drink yourself to death but I cannot allow you to freeze to death". The man died a fortnight later and in his will he left "To my friend, Dr William Osler, his overcoat and my hob-nailed liver".

A few examples of his well-known sayings may be quoted:

"A student practitioner requires three things — a note book, a library and a quinquennial brain-dusting".

"The value of experience is not in seeing much but in seeing wisely".

"Look wise, say nothing and grunt. Speech was given to conceal thought".

"One swallow does not make a summer but one tophus makes gout and one crescent malaria".

Osler had an irrepressible tendency to play practical jokes for some of which he assumed the name of Egerton Y. Davis who lived in a fictitious town called Caughnawuga. Many honours came to Osler, including the F.R.S. in 1898 and a baronetcy in 1911. He gave several of the commemorative lectures at the Royal College of Physicians and its Harveian Oration. The brotherhood of medicine was his ideal and this accounts for his activity in the founding of the Association of Physicians in 1907. In 1892 Osler married Grace Revere Gross, the widow of his friend Samuel W. Gross. It is recorded that even on his honeymoon he could not be kept away from medical meetings.

As well as having an omnivorous curiosity Osler was blessed with a charm of personality and buoyancy of spirit. These qualities, with his kindness and lack of malice, made him the ideal physician. He was certainly a master of the clinical art and had a greater influence on the English-speaking medical world of his day on both sides of the Atlantic than anyone else. Optimism and equanimity were his watchwords and he said that a nature "sloping towards the southern side" helped greatly in the practice of medicine. It may have helped him to bear the deep sorrow which came to him in 1917 when his only son, Edward Revere Osler, was killed at Ypres, for he bore it with the equanimity he had taught. The strain, however, must have contributed to his death on 29th December 1919 in Oxford.

Osler gave his own library to the medical school at McGill and there his ashes lie. Having done his most important teaching in the wards he suggested as his epitaph: "I taught medicine at the bedside".

PAGET'S DISEASE OF BONE
PAGET'S DISEASE OF THE NIPPLE
Sir James Paget Bt 1814-1889

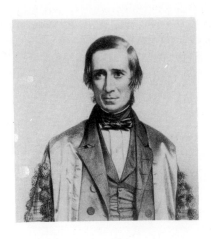

JAMES PAGET is remembered for his original descriptions of two conditions which are still referred to in his name and are both so perfect that virtually nothing has been added to them since from the clinical side. Paget's disease of the nipple, a pre-cancerous condition, was described in 1874. Paget's disease of bone, described in 1877, used to be called osteitis deformans but as it is not an inflammatory condition a better term would be osteo-dystrophia deformans. But "deformans" only applies to a few cases and many are clinically insignificant and only shown by x-rays.

This great surgeon was born in Great Yarmouth on 11th January 1814, the youngest of the nine surviving children from 17 born to Samuel and Sarah Paget. He attended a school in Yarmouth but had to leave when aged 13 because his father's business as a brewer and ship-owner began to fail. He was greatly attracted to botany of which he said: "The knowledge was useless;

the discipline of acquiring it beyond all price". He published "The Natural History of Great Yarmouth" when aged 20. At 16 he had been apprenticed to Charles Costerton, a surgeon-apothecary in Yarmouth. In 1834 he became a student at St Bartholomew's Hospital, his fees being paid by his elder brother, George. While still a student there he discovered that the gritty particles commonly seen in muscles were the encysted larvae of the worm *Trichinella spiralis*. The teaching at St Bartholomew's was poor in those days but James worked hard on his own account and obtained the qualification M.R.C.S. in 1836. He had a hard struggle to maintain himself and was engaged to Lydia North for seven years before he could afford to marry her. He said his engagement gave him "help and hope to make even the heaviest work seem light". He took a pupil for a time and was sub-editor of the London Gazette. He earned a little for translating and reviewing books and reporting lectures. As curator of the museum at St Bartholomew's Hospital he was paid £40 a year. When he lived in two rooms over the wig-maker's shop at 3 Searle Street, Lincoln's Inn Fields, his practice brought him £13 or £14 a year, his total income being £170. He gave up journalism when he became warden of the students' residential college and was then able to marry. He was one of the 300 original Fellows of the Royal College of Surgeons when it became "of England" in 1843 (having been "of London" when it was founded in 1800) and was its professor of anatomy.

Paget became assistant surgeon to St Bartholomew's Hospital at 33. When 38 he was in practice at 24 Henrietta Street, Cavendish Square, and rapidly rose to the top of his profession. When he looked after the Princess of Wales people began to hear about him and by 1878 he was earning £10,000 a year. But he was very modest about this and remarked that "mere notoriety in some people's minds is a sign of merit". He then gave up operating and restricted himself to consultations. He had worked extremely hard and only took his first holiday in 1861, the reason being that he was determined to pay off the heavy debts left by his father. He was surgeon-extraordinary to Queen Victoria for 41 years and a great friend of the Royal Family.

In 1871 he had "blood poisoning" acquired when doing a post-mortem. This severe illness caused him to give up active hospital work but his private consulting practice continued. A baronetcy was conferred on him. He held many important positions: president of the Royal College of Surgeons, member of the General Medical Council and member of the Senate of the University of London and its vice-chancellor. He worked hard till the end of his life and said: "There is no true success without work". In 1894 he moved to 4 Park Square West but did not practise there. He was one of the few medical men who up to the end of the 19th century have written autobiographies. Paget died on 30th December 1889, a few days before his 80th birthday. He was buried in Finchley cemetery after a funeral service in Westminster Abbey.

Paget was tall and slim with a sensitive intellectual face and bright eyes. He had a beautiful voice and was a fine orator. Henry Parr, the great ophthalmic surgeon, wrote that he was "a very winning lecturer altogether, the best I ever heard". A man quite free from envy and uncharitableness, he showed universal courtesy and generosity and was one of the great Victorians. One of his sons became Bishop of Oxford and another, Stephen Paget, was a well-known surgeon and author of Confessio Medici.

PARKINSON'S DISEASE
James Parkinson 1755-1824

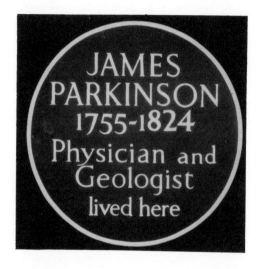

"AN essay on the Shaking Palsy" was written by James Parkinson, Member of the Royal College of Surgeons, at the age of 62 and was published in London in 1817 as a slim volume of 66 pages. Long recognised as one of the minor classics of medicine, this little book was never reprinted and is now exceedingly rare. The essential part of Parkinson's description runs as follows:

> "*Shaking palsy (paralysis agitans). Involuntary tremulous motion, with lessened muscular power, in parts not in action and even when supported: with a propensity to bend the trunk forward and to pass from a walking to a running pace: the senses and intellect being uninjured*".

Although Parkinson dealt with only six cases, two of which were "casually met with in the street" and another only "seen at a distance", he gave an excellent description of the clinical features of the disease and separated it from a group of maladies showing weakness and tremor. He omitted, however, to mention the bradykinesia so characteristic of the disease. Charcot added this some 40 years later and proposed the name Parkinson's Disease. This became a fully established eponym from the time of the world epidemic of encephalitis lethargica around 1920.

James Parkinson was born on 11th April 1755, the son of John Parkinson, apothecary and surgeon (the equivalent of the present general practitioner), of 1 Hoxton Square, London, at that time a most desirable locality. He spent all his life in the East End of London, being baptised, married (in 1781) and buried (in 1824) in St Leonard's Church, Shoreditch. He was for six months a pupil of Richard Grindall F.R.S., assistant surgeon to the London Hospital, and his name appears in the list of approved surgeons of the Corporation of Surgeons of London in 1784. He was always an opponent of the apprenticeship system of medical education and felt that a period of training in hospital was necessary. In 1785 he found time to attend John Hunter's lectures and took shorthand notes which were published posthumously in 1893 by his eldest son, T. W. K. Parkinson F.R.C.S., under the title, "Hunterian Reminiscences". James later inherited his father's house and practice and so adhered to the tradition of those days by which an eldest son followed the profession or trade of his father. Another reason may have been financial, as he probably had ambitions for consultant work for which he was certainly fitted. He is known to have commented in later life: "A physician seldom obtains bread by his profession until he has no teeth left to eat it".

Parkinson was a man of great intellectual activity and his interests extended far beyond the bounds of what might have been expected of a busy general practitioner. His contemporary reputation rested on his geological works of which the *magnum opus*, "Organic remains of a former world", appeared in three volumes in 1804, 1808 and 1811. This work was beautifully illustrated by large plates and formed a landmark in the history of palaentology. The ancient term for palaentology was oryctology and Parkinson's treatise, "Outlines of Oryctology", appeared in 1822. He made a large collection of fossils and was an original member of the Geological Society of London and an honorary member of the Imperial Society of Natural History of St Petersburg.

There was much political unrest in Parkinson's time and he, an ardent radical, wrote tracts or "penny pamphlets" on political and social reform such as "Revolution without bloodshed or Revolution preferable to revolt" (1794). He belonged to several political secret societies including the London Corresponding Society for which he wrote under the pen-name of Old Hubert. In 1794 some members of this society were charged with complicity in an alleged plot to kill King George III. It was planned to create a diversion at the theatre "by quarrels, combats and cries of Pickpockets" so that when the King leaned forward in his box to see what was going on he would present a target for a poisoned arrow discharged from a popgun. Those accused in this "popgun plot" were thrown into prison and detained for months without trial. Parkinson, who was subpoenaed but not called, wrote a pamphlet, "A vindication of the Corresponding Society", maintaining its innocence and clamouring against the suspension of the Habeas Corpus Act. In October 1794 he gave evidence on oath before the Privy Council where he had a long verbal duel with the Attorney General. Parkinson dropped politics at the age of 40 and concentrated on medicine and his hobby of palaentology. Another of his interests was health education of lay people. "Medical admonitions to families" appeared in 1799 and in "The Villager's Friend and Physician", 1800, he represents himself as an old village apothecary who is retiring after 30 years' practice and who gives some parting advice to his old patients. "Dangerous Sports, a cautionary tale for children" appeared in 1800.

Like Sydenham he suffered from gout and in 1805 he wrote his "Observations on the Nature and Cure of Gout". Parkinson helped his son to report the first case of appendicitis recorded in British medical literature. The paper, entitled "A case of diseased appendix vermiformis" (Medico-Chirurgical Transactions 1816 3 57), describes a fatal case in a boy of five. Many of his ideas about training in medicine are stated in "The Hospital Pupil" which consists of four letters he wrote in 1800. One piece of advice in it about reading is: "Never read but with your pen in your hand and your commonplace book beside you, in which you will enter such passages as strike your mind by their novelty and importance".

Parkinson is described by his friend Gideon Mantell as being in later life "rather below the middle stature, with an energetic, intelligent and pleasing countenance and of mild and courteous manners readily imparting information of his favourite subjects". The honours that came to him were mostly for his palaeontological work but in 1822 he was the first recipient of the gold medal of the Royal College of Surgeons. Parkinson married Mary Dale on 21st May 1781 when he was 26 and they had two sons and two daughters.

When his busy and honourable life ended on 21st December 1824 the medical profession did nothing to commemorate him, perhaps because of his political views. Dr Leonard Rowntree, an American historian, rescued him from oblivion by an article in which he said of him: "English born, English bred, forgotten by the English and by the world at large, such was the fate of James Parkinson" (Bulletin of the Johns Hopkins Hospital 1912 23 33). No portrait of Parkinson has ever been found*. This omission was repaired to some extent by the memorial plaque provided by the governors of The London Hospital and unveiled on 31st August 1961 at the furniture factory of Lewis Wolf and Sons, 1 Hoxton Square, Shoreditch, London, on the site of Parkinson's birthplace. Another memorial tablet was placed in St Leonard's Church by the nursing staff of St Leonard's Hospital on 17th September 1955. No stone bearing his name exists in the churchyard.

Parkinson was not a brilliant investigator and he made no startling contribution to medicine. But he was a great compilator and a keen observer who liked to have everything named and in its proper class. He accurately described a disease which has made his name one of the most used eponyms.

---

*One supposedly of him and published in America (Medical Classics 1937-38 vol 2 937) proved to be that of a dentist of the same name taken at a meeting of the British Dental Association. The dentist was wearing clothes fashionable 100 years after Parkinson's time.

PAUL'S TUBE
Frank Thomas Paul 1851-1941

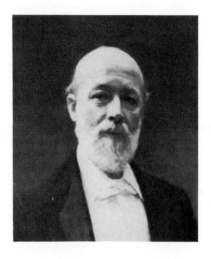

BEFORE Paul's time faecal leakage made excision of portions of the large bowel dangerous. Glass tubes connected to rubber tubing eliminated this risk and Paul described their use in a paper "A new method of performing inguinal colostomy" (British Medical Journal 1891 2 118). Since then his tubes have been used all over the world. He is remembered also for his method of extra-abdominal resection of the colon — sometimes referred to as the Paul-Mikulicz operation.

Frank Paul was born on 3rd December 1851 at Ashwood Lodge, Pentney, Norfolk. His early education was at Downham and Lynn with a final year when aged 15, at Yarmouth Grammar School. After leaving school he found work in a broker's office in London very dull and begged to be allowed to study medicine. Apprenticeship to a local physician had to be terminated, however, as his master was not a licentiate of the Society of Apothecaries. So Paul went to Guy's Hospital where he lived in the quadrangle. He records that it took him weeks to become hardened to operations and post-mortems. By the age of 22 he had qualified L.S.A. and M.R.C.S. and soon after was L.R.C.P. also, and had passed the primary examination for the F.R.C.S.

House posts for 18 months were followed by appointment as resident medical officer at the Liverpool Royal Infirmary in 1875. Here he found the staff excellent though the custom was still to operate in dirty old pre-Listerian frock coats. After eight years he became surgeon to the Stanley Hospital while retaining the post of pathologist to the Royal Infirmary. He practised at 38 Rodney Street but private patients were few and he lived largely on his fees from giving anaesthetics. After five years' work at the Stanley Hospital he became surgeon to the Royal Southern Hospital and there developed his interest in abdominal surgery. In 1891 he was elected surgeon to the Liverpool Royal Infirmary where he worked until he reached the age limit 20 years later. It was a wonderful period during which the safety of operations increased astoundingly. Patients lost their dread of the operating theatre and were often caused more distress by being refused an operation than by being recommended for one.

Paul was prominent in fields other than abdominal surgery and by 1897 had done partial thyroidectomy in six cases of exophthalmic goitre without a death. In his lifetime he amputated the breast for cancer 1,000 times without a death. He took an active part in the work of the Medical School both before and after its incorporation as the Medical Faculty of the University of Liverpool. He served throughout the First World War at the 2nd Western General Hospital at Fazakerly, on the outskirts of Liverpool. After retirement from the Royal Infirmary he continued to work at Hoylake Cottage Hospital and did not give up surgery entirely until he was 80.

Paul had a highly sensitive nature and his gentleness in handling tissues attracted the attention of visiting surgeons. A result of this was the presentation to the Liverpool Medical Institution by his colleague, Frank Jeans, of a bronze cast of his right hand. In the presentation speech Jeans said: "Paul operating in the hey-day of his career always made me think that he did with his hands what Pavlova did with her feet, only Paul's work was much more useful". In his reply Paul reminded Jeans that "the gentle touch comes from the heart rather than from the hands".

Matters other than practical surgery claimed a good deal of Paul's time and he was professor of medical jurisprudence for several years though never professor of surgery. He was for a time dean of the faculty of medicine. But his first love was the Medical Institution in Liverpool to which he was greatly attached and of which he was president in 1906-07.

Having been nurtured in the country, Paul always felt its call, though opportunities for hunting and fishing were few when he came north. In his Liverpool days he was a canoeing and camping enthusiast. He married in 1888 Geraldine, a nursing sister at the Royal Southern Hospital and daughter of Eustace Gregg and a cousin of William Rathbone, a pioneer of nursing reform. They had three daughters. His country home was at Hoylake and later at Caldy in the Wirral but he retired to Grayshott, near Hindhead, Surrey to be near his children and to grow orchids. He died there on 17th January 1941, aged 89. Paul was a modest and self-effacing man of fine presence with a full beard.

POTT'S FRACTURE
POTT'S DISEASE
Percivall Pott 1714-1788

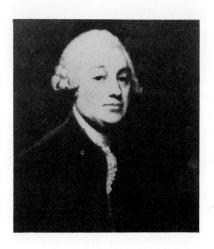

IN January 1755 Percivall Pott was thrown from his horse in the Old Kent Road and sustained a compound fracture of the tibia. Being well aware of the dangers of rough handling he would not allow himself to be moved until he had sent for two chair men. He purchased a back door and, when the chair men's poles were nailed to it, he was carried over London Bridge to Watling Street, a tremendous distance for a man in his state. It is of interest that he chose not to be taken to Guy's Hospital which was only 400 yards away. Amputation was advised by many of his fellow surgeons and Pott accepted their opinion and the instruments were got ready. But Pott was saved from operation by his old teacher, Edward Nourse, who arrived late at the consultation. He conceived the idea of preserving the limb. After reduction the position of the exit of the bone through the skin was at a distance from the break in the bone so that the intervening tissues formed a sort of valve which excluded the air. During his convalescence

Pott planned his Treatise on Ruptures.

Percivall Pott was born on 6th January 1714 in a house on a site in Threadneedle Street in the City of London where the Bank of England now stands. His father, a scrivener or drafter of documents, died when Percivall was only three-years-old. Percivall was sent to a private school at Darenth in Kent until he was 15. He was then apprenticed to Edward Nourse, assistant surgeon to St Bartholomew's Hospital, the fee of 200 guineas being paid by a wealthy relative, the Bishop of Rochester.

In 1736 he obtained the diploma of the Barber Surgeons' Company. He first practised in Fenchurch Street where he lived with his mother and sister. In 1745, when Nourse became full surgeon, Pott was made assistant surgeon. Soon after the death of his mother in 1745 Percivall married Sarah Cruttenden and they moved to a house in Watling Street. Here he gave lectures on anatomy and surgery. In 1749 he became surgeon to St Bartholomew's Hospital where he stood out as a giant among the members of the staff. He was the virtual founder of the medical school there. He practised in Princess Street, Hanover Square, where he enjoyed the largest, most fashionable and most lucrative practice in London. This enabled him to educate his large family of nine children. He also had a house at Neasden, Middlesex. He received many honours, including Fellowship of the .Royal Society in 1765.

The eponymously named Pott's fracture is not the one he sustained himself but a fracture of the fibula with dislocation of the ankle. This was described in a book, "Some few general remarks on Fractures and Dislocations", by Percivall Pott F.R.S., 1769. Pott's disease of the spine or tuberculosis of a vertebra was described in 1779. In the first edition of his book on head injuries he refers to a "puffy tumour" of the scalp which is caused by oedema overlying osteomyelitis. It is not a tumour in the neoplastic sense, the word being, with calor, dolor and rubor, an indication of inflammation.

Pott was a wise teacher of surgery who decried the cult of speed, saying:

"Time has produced a most absurd custom of measuring the motion of a surgeon's hands as jockeys do that of the feet of a

horse, viz: by a stopwatch, a practice which, though it may
perhaps have been encouraged by operators themselves, must
have been productive of most mischievous consequences . . .
as the operator has no recompense from the reputation which
the latter obtains from the bystanders".

Pott's appearance is described as "elegant, lower than middle size". He was always neatly dressed and had a youthful appearance until the end of his life. He was a man of honesty and integrity and often gave some of his handsome income to the unfortunate. He died of pneumonia, contracted on making a 20 mile journey to see a patient. As he lay dying he said: "My life is almost extinguished. I hope it has burned for the benefit of others". He was buried in the church of St Mary Aldermary in the City of London where there is a commemorative tablet. The obituary notice in The Annual Register 1788 page 24 says:

"He was an interesting converser; he had cultivated
literature; he was fond of art. But his best praise was in real
life in the relative duties and more trying efforts of active life.
In the more pecuniary parts of character happy is he who can
be as liberal".

RAMSTEDT'S OPERATION
Conrad Ramstedt 1867-1963

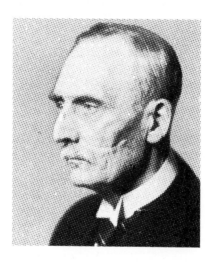

HYPERTROPHIC pyloric stenosis in infants had been described in 1888 by Harald Hirschprung but, as pyloroplasty for its relief usually ended fatally, physicians were reluctant to advise it. Ramstedt first performed his operation on 23rd August 1911 and several different accounts of it have been given. Ramstedt's own description is to be found in a letter dated 30th July 1957 to Dr W. F. Pollock of Los Angeles ("Dr Conrad Ramstedt and pylorotomy" by W. H. Pollock and W. J. Norris, Surgery 1957 42 966). The patient was the first-born son of a distinguished and noble family and the first case of the condition Ramstedt had seen.

"At the laparotomy on 23rd August 1911 I was astonished at the pyloric tumour as thick as my thumb. After I had split the tumour down to the mucosa for a distance of about 2 cm I had the impression that the stenosis had been relieved. I still tried, however, to accomplish the plastic procedure by transverse

suture of the muscle edges. However, the tension on the sutures was so very strong that the first ·one cut through immediately. Then the thought shot through my head: 'A plastic alteration of the cut edges is completely unnecessary; the stenosis seems to be already relieved by the simple splitting of the pyloric muscle and coincidentally the spasm as well, which is the characteristic basis of the disease'.

I did not complete the plastic operation on the muscle which had been originally planned but left the cut gaping, covering it with a tab of omentum for safety's sake and ended the operation. The little one vomited a few times for the first few days, which I attributed to the sutures placed at the beginning, but he recovered promptly and completely to the great joy of his parents".

The operation was successfully performed for a second time on 18th June 1912 when the incision was deliberately left gaping without any attempt at suture. The child was the son of a physician and it is remarkable that nearly all the early patients of Ramstedt's large series were children of medical men. Ramstedt reported his first two cases to the Natural Sciences Assembly at Münster (Medizinische Klinik 1912 8 1702 and Zentralblatt für Chirurgie 1913 40 3). Since that time the mortality has fallen from 50 per cent to around one per cent and Ramstedt's procedure has proved to be the most consistently successful operation ever devised.

Conrad Ramstedt, the son of a physician, was born at Hamersleben, a village in Central Prussia. He attended the gymnasium at Magdeburg and studied medicine at Heidelburg, Berlin and Halle, graduating M.D. Halle in 1894. From 1895 to 1901 he was assistant in the surgical clinic there and then became a military surgeon. He held high rank in the medical department of the German Army during the 1914-18 war and in 1919 became the chief surgeon to the Rafaelklinik at Münster. As well as five articles on the surgical treatment of pyloric stenosis he also wrote the chapters on surgery of the male genito-urinary organs in the Handbuch der praktischen Chirurgie, edited by Bergman and Mikulicz and published in 1927.

Ramstedt was a connoisseur of art and made a special study of the Dutch masters. His younger daughter is a well-known sculptress, Tita Tork-Ramstedt. Ramstedt died on 7th February 1963 at the age of 95 after a fruitful life during which he had the rare experience of seeing his own contribution to surgery accepted universally.

Students of surgical history will have noticed that in the original account of his operation the author spelt his name Rammstedt but that in later papers it appeared as Ramstedt. When he was inquiring into his own genealogy he was surprised to find that his grandfather had made an error in his entry in the church records. It is thought that nervousness at his wedding caused him to sign his name with two "m"s. In 1920 Ramstedt changed the spelling to conform to earlier records. His daughter also made the change but his son still used the form with two "m"s.

RAYNAUD'S DISEASE
Maurice Raynaud 1834-1881

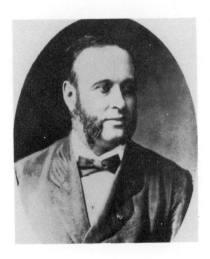

A GRADUATION thesis, once it has served its immediate purpose, is usually soon forgotten but that of Maurice Raynaud for the degree of M.D. in 1862, "On local asphyxia and symmetrical gangrene of the extremities", was an exception. It gave Raynaud's name a place in every textbook of medicine; it was supplemented in 1884 and both memoirs were published in English in 1888 by the New Sydenham Society among their selected monographs. The translator and editor was Dr (later Sir) Thomas Barlow, the father of the profession in England. He records that Raynaud's work was brought before English readers by Dr Reginald Southey in St Bartholomew's Hospital Reports 1880 and, about the same time, by Mr (later Sir) Johnathan Hutchinson in his Hunterian lectures at the Royal College of Surgeons.

Raynaud accepted credit for the description of a new disease but would not speculate on its pathological features, saying:
"I do not aspire to the frivolous and dangerous honour of

making an innovation in pathology. To describe a new disease, and especially to give a new name to a group of symptoms which have long been observed and described, is assuredly less difficult than to link together, under a common law which dominates them, many affections apparently different".

Raynaud's disease may be defined as "intermittent pallor or cyanosis of the extremities brought on by cold, with the skin a normal colour between attacks". The essential part of Raynaud's description of the severe form of the disease reads as follows:

"I propose to demonstrate that there exists a variety of dry gangrene affecting the extremities which it is impossible to explain by a vascular obliteration, a variety characterised especially by a remarkable tendency to symmetry, so that it always affects similar parts, the two upper or lower limbs or the four at the same time, further, in certain cases, the nose and the ears; and I hope to prove that this kind of gangrene has its cause in a vice of innervation of the capillary vessels which it remains for me to define".

Unfortunately, Raynaud included descriptions of cases in his original and subsequent reports which were not representative of the syndrome.

Maurice Raynaud was born on 10th August 1834, the son of a distinguished university professor. He began his medical studies under the auspices of his uncle, A. G. M. Vernois (1809-1977), an eminent physician in Paris. He received his doctor's degree in 1862. In addition to his famous thesis Raynaud also wrote a thesis on Asclepiades of Bithynia and also an account of physicians in the time of Molière (1622-1673). For these scholarly works he obtained his licence (doctor's degree) in letters. With these brilliant achievements a senior appointment might have been expected but he never achieved it. Raynaud was never offered a senior post though his great ambition was to hold the chair of Medical History in Paris; this was denied him, it is said, because of his activity in the Roman Catholic Church. He became physician to the hospitals in 1863 and was attached at various times to the Hôtel-Dieu, the Lariboisière and the Charité hospitals. He was made an officer of the Legion of Honour in 1871 and was elected to the Académie de Médicine in 1879. He was selected to deliver the address in medicine at the International Medical Congress in London in 1881 but died suddenly on 30th June a few days before he should have travelled to England. He had suffered from organic heart disease for many years. His address on "Scepticism in medicine past and present" was read to the Congress by one of his colleagues. Raynaud was a man of spotless character, absolute integrity and great intellectual achievements.

REITER'S DISEASE
Hans Conrad Reiter 1881-1969

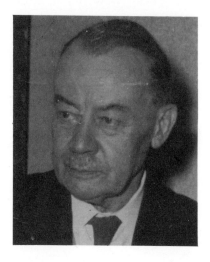

WHEN he was serving on the Balkan front with the first Hungarian Army during the 1914-18 war Reiter looked after a young lieutenant suffering from a triad of symptoms — urethritis, conjunctivitis and arthritis. At first he considered it to be due to a spirochaetal infection and he called it spirochaetosis arthritica but, as salvarsan did not affect it, he soon retracted this view. The condition has since been called Reiter's disease although a full account of five cases had been given in 1818 by Sir Benjamin Brodie (1783-1862) in his textbook, "Diseases of the Bones and Joints". Reiter focused attention on a new aspect of the condition — its association with dysentery — and initiated a period of research into its problems which persists to the present day.

Hans Reiter was born in Leipzig in 1881, the son of an industrialist. He attended the gymnasium and began studying medicine at the age of 20, first in Leipzig and then in Breslau and

Tübingen. He gained his M.D. with a dissertation on "Nephritis and tuberculosis". Then followed a period of experience abroad — in Paris, London and Berlin. He worked under Sir Almroth Wright at St Mary's Hospital, London for two years. In 1913 he was appointed *privat-dozent* (or recognised teacher) at the Institute of Hygiene, Königsberg, and for a few months preceding the 1914-18 war he was deputy director at the Institute of Hygiene in the University of Berlin. While serving on the Western Front in the 1914-18 war he identified the causative organism of Weil's disease, a feat which had eluded others for many years. His next discovery was the condition which bears his name. Another achievement was the isolation of a non-pathogenic cultivable variant of *Treponema pallidum* which later provided an antigen for a highly specific test for treponemal disease — the Reiter complement fixation test.

After the war Reiter was made professor of hygiene at Rostock University and this was followed by his appointment in 1933 as a section director at the Kaiser Wilhelm Institute of Experimental Therapy in Berlin-Dahlem. Three years later he became director of the health department of the State of Mecklenburg. He was politically active and became a follower of Adolf Hitler, partly on account of his theoretical interest in eugenics. He signed an oath of allegiance to Hitler in 1932 and so he received appointments under the Nazi government — president of the health department of Berlin and honorary professor.

Reiter had enormous vitality and as an octogenarian, he presented a paper at the International Congress on Rheumatism in Rome. His work was not only in the laboratory; he was very active in the field of applied hygiene and, as well as being a researcher, he was a brilliant teacher. He received the Robert Koch medal and the Great Medal of Honour of the Red Cross. He was an affiliate member of the Royal Society of London. In later years he studied the many problems of the illegitimate child. A tall, dignified figure with an innate courtesy characteristic of an age now passed, he lived after retirement in his country house at Kassel-Wilhelmshoe, Hessen, where he died on 25th November 1969 at the age of 88.

THE ARGYLL ROBERTSON PUPIL
Douglas Argyll Robertson 1837-1909

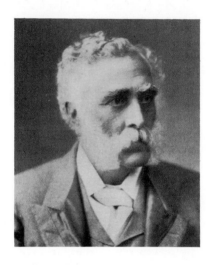

ARGYLL ROBERTSON's full name — Douglas Moray Cooper Lamb Argyll Robertson — was only revealed in his obituaries, as he always signed himself D. Argyll Robertson. He is universally known by the eponym, the Argyll Robertson pupil, and was the first surgeon in Scotland to practise entirely in the field of ophthalmology. His father, John Argyll Robertson, who became president of the Royal College of Surgeons of Edinburgh in 1848, was a general surgeon but specially interested in the eye and one of the founders of the Edinburgh Eye Dispensary. Two of his uncles were Fellows of the College. Douglas was born in 1837. He began his medical studies in Edinburgh but graduated M.D. from St Andrew's in 1857 when he was 20. After being house surgeon at the Edinburgh Royal Infirmary he studied under Albrecht von Graefe in Berlin. On his return to Edinburgh he taught a laboratory class in physiology while developing his practice in ophthalmology. In 1867 he was made assistant ophthalmic surgeon to the Royal Infirmary, becoming full ophthalmic surgeon in 1870.

In July 1868 a 50-year-old tailor, George Smith, felt giddy when crossing the North Bridge in Edinburgh and next day his legs felt numb. By December he was complaining about his eyes and Argyll Robertson, who saw him, reported: "On examination, I found that while walking his gait was unsteady and that he could not plant his feet firmly on the ground. On looking at the eyes, the drooping of the lids and the small pupils at once attracted attention. The drooping of the lids was more marked in the left than in the right eye — the left palpebral aperture at the widest point measuring only 3.3/4 lines while the right measured 4 lines. Each pupil measured three-quarters of a line in diameter; they were insensible to the influence of light but contracted to half a line during the act of accommodation for a near object".

The patient had tabes dorsalis and a study of five similar patients made Robertson conclude that for contraction of the pupil under light it is necessary that the cilio-spinal nerves remained intact and that when, as in the case of miosis, the cilio-spinal nerves are paralysed, light does not influence the pupil. The Argyll Robertson pupil which reacts to accommodation but not to light almost always indicates syphilis of the central nervous system. Its description was given in a paper, "On an Interesting Series of Eye Symptoms in a case of Spinal Disease with remarks on the Action of Belladonna on the Iris, etc. (Edinburgh Medical Journal 1869 14 696). The condition is usually permanent but a few examples of pupils returning to normal after anti-syphilitic treatment have been reported.

Argyll Robertson made major contributions to ophthalmic surgery. He searched for a drug which would have the opposite effect to atropine and stimulate the sphincter pupillae. At the suggestion of his friend, Thomas R. Fraser, he did experiments on himself with extracts of Calabar bean *(Physostigma venenosum)*. Its active ingredient (later shown to be eserine or physostigmine) contracted the ciliary muscle of accommodation and the sphincter pupillae, both being supplied by the ciliary nerves.

Argyll Robertson was a tall, handsome man whose frock coat and top hat gave him an air of distinction which, with his old-world courtesy, endeared him to his colleagues and patients. He shunned controversy but, if he had to enter upon it, he was a resolute and skilful, but always kind, antagonist. He was specially concerned for the honour of his profession. He always did what he could to "save face" for anyone who had unwittingly made an error in diagnosis or treatment. In 1886 he became president of the Royal College of Surgeons of Edinburgh and was the first president of the Ophthalmic Society who did not practise in London. He married in 1882 but, having no children, he and his wife undertook the education of Prince and Princess Taraba, the children of the Thakur of Gondal who had been one of Argyll Robertson's students.

Argyll Robertson retired in 1904 to a farm, Mon Plaisir, at St Aubins, Jersey. He was very fond of social life, a member of many clubs and a polished after-dinner speaker. A great golfer, he was wont to say: "Of all recreations commend me to golf", which he regarded as the best of all. He won the gold medal of the Royal and Ancient Club at St Andrew's five times. He died, aged 72, on 3rd January 1909 when on his third visit to India. His body was cremated on the bank of the river Gondhi.

ROMBERG'S SIGN
Moritz Heinrich Romberg 1795-1873

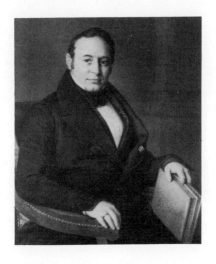

By relating altered structure to clinical manifestations, Romberg's "Lehrbuch der Nervenkrankheiten des Menschen" (1849) represented the first successful attempt to write a comprehensive treatise on nervous diseases. Although his nosology was slowly abandoned as specific neurological entities were recognised, his fame rests on his success in being the first to bring order into neurological thought. In his epoch-making work Romberg considered the earlier literature of neurology, gave clear-cut clinical pictures and attempted to systematize a group of diseases that had hitherto received little attention. He derived much of the background of his work from Sir Charles Bell's "The Nervous System of the Human Body" (1830) and stated: "The researches of Sir Charles Bell fill me with enthusiasm and in 1831 I translated his great work and made known to my professional brethren in Germany his investigations which will ever serve as models of scientific inquiry". In the second edition of his own work (1851 vol 2 p 185) Romberg described his own well-known sign that patients with locomotor ataxia cannot stand with their eyes shut: "Lässt man in aufrechter Stellung die Augen schliessen, so fängt er sofort an zu schwanken und zu taumeln . . ." (If one lets him close his eyes standing he immediately begins to sway and to stumble). I called attention to this pathognomonic sign ten years ago (according to my observation it does not occur either in other paralyses or in uncomplicated illness) and have since never failed to find it in any of my numerous patients with this disease". At a time when the horse was a common means of transport it is interesting to record that Romberg said: "The rider no longer feels the resistance of the stirrup and has the strap put up a hole or two".

Romberg's name is also joined with that of John Howship (died 1841) in the Romberg-Howship sign. This refers to the lancinating pains in the leg which occur in incarcerated obturator hernia. He described it in the third edition of his treatise (1843-57, p. 89). Facial hemiatrophy, which is sometimes called Romberg's disease, was described by the great neurologist in his "Klinische Ergebnisse" in 1846.

Moritz Heinrich Romberg, the son of a merchant, was born at Meiningen, capital of the former Duchy of Saxe-Meiningen (now just inside the border of East Germany), on 11th November 1795. He studied medicine in Berlin and took his doctor's degree in 1817 with a thesis on "congenital rickets" (it contained a classic description of achondroplasia). After graduation he spent some time in Vienna where he enjoyed the friendship of Dr John Peter Frank, the celebrated writer on public health. On his return to Berlin he was appointed (1820) as one of the official physicians of the poor and in 1830 he became *privat-dozent* (or recognised teacher) of special pathology and therapeutics. He acted as director of a cholera hospital during the epidemics of 1831 and 1837. In 1834 he turned his private hospital into a kind of postgraduate clinic where he excelled as a teacher of methods of physical diagnosis. Appointed extraordinary professor in 1838, he became director of the Berlin University Clinic in 1840 and an ordinary professor of special pathology and therapeutics in 1845. He was made a geheim-medizinal-rath in 1851 and when he celebrated the 50th jubilee of his doctorate 29th March 1867 his fame was world-wide. Romberg died of heart disease on 16th June 1873. The great neurologist was an uncle of Eduard Henoch, of Henoch's purpura.

RYLE'S TUBE
John Ryle 1889-1950

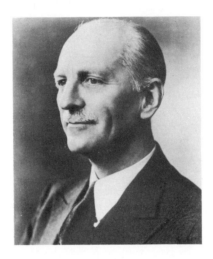

RYLE's tube is used every day in many general hospitals and is well-known to every doctor and nurse, but it commemorates only one phase in the varied life of Professor Ryle. John Alfred Ryle was born in 1889, the third in a family of ten children of Dr J. R. Ryle, of Brighton. He was educated at Brighton College and at Guy's Hospital where he qualified in 1913 and won the gold medal in medicine. While serving in the Royal Army Medical Corps he investigated typhoid and trench fever. After the first World War he made his mark as an outstanding and eloquent teacher at Guy's Hospital. He spent his weekends in studying the gastric juice, which he obtained through a large (Einhorn) tube with a brass terminal fitting. It was his wife's failure to swallow the original tube which made her suggest that a smaller all-rubber tube would do equally well and so it was that Ryle's tube was born (Guy's Hospital Reports, 1921, 71, 22).

Ryle's interest in symptoms was that of a naturalist and so he studied the course which diseases took when unaltered by treatment. Much of his original thinking is recorded in "The Natural History of Disease", published in 1936. His academic turn of'mind, and perhaps the heavy strain of his huge practice in London, made him take the opportunity in 1935, at the early age of 46, to become regius professor of physic at Cambridge, a mainly administrative post. While at Cambridge he surveyed all the hospitals near the East Coast from Newcastle to London to decide which could be used as emergency hospitals in the event of war.

When war did break out he worked in the Emergency Medical Service. He was pleased, however, to return to Guy's to help to maintain the standard of teaching and patient care which had fallen off when many consultants joined the forces. When he became consultant adviser to the Minister of Health he gave up his chair at Cambridge where he had never been really happy. In 1943 he found scope for his idealism in the newly-created post of professor of social medicine at Oxford. Here he studied the effect of environmental factors in the production of disease and, in spite of poor health, travelled widely. His firm advocacy of a National Health Service and less disparity between the status of consultants and other doctors led to incomprehension and hostility from many of his colleagues. Perhaps because he was an idealist and had some of the idealist's limitations, certain of his projects were only partially successful. The move to social medicine was to him the logical conclusion of a life-long interest in studying the cause of disease. It also satisfied his social conscience and his desire to do more for the underprivileged. His years at Oxford were probably his happiest. Ryle's prestige in the profession was probably a factor which secured recognition of social medicine at Oxford. Ryle was a tall and handsome man. A great teacher, he was utterly honest and always kind.

SCARPA'S TRIANGLE
Antonio Scarpa 1747-1832

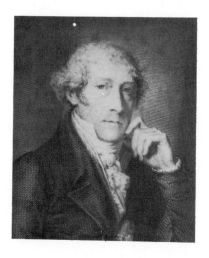

SCARPA's name has been attached in the past to several anatomical structures. The best known eponym, Scarpa's triangle commemorates one of his lesser contributions to anatomical knowledge.

Scarpa was born at Lorenzaga, in the commune of Motta di Livenza, on the southern slopes of the mountains lying between Northern Italy and Austria. The date was 19th May and the year is variously given as 1747, 1748 and 1752. His father, Guiseppe Scarpa, was a small tradesman of Venetian origin. Nothing is known of Scarpa's early life except that his education was undertaken by his uncle Don Paolo, a priest. He went to the University of Padua at the age of 15 and there attracted the attention of Morgagni, the old and almost blind professor of anatomy. He had the inestimable privilege of acting as his personal secretary — a great training in itself, for he wrote Morgagni's replies to requests for opinions on cases which reached him from all over Europe. Two years at Padua were followed by two at Bologna and then in 1770 Scarpa returned to Padua to take his doctor's degree. He was elected professor of anatomy at Modena at the early age of 22 and taught there for eight years In 1780 he made the first of three scientific journeys to centres of learning in England, France, Germany and Austria. In London he worked under Percivall Pott, William and John Hunter and William Cruikshank. On his return he was made professor of anatomy at Padua (1783) and remained there for the rest of his life.

Throughout the tumultuous times of the French Revolutionary Wars Scarpa worked in his dissecting room, but when the Transpaduan Republic was proclaimed in 1796 he refused to take the oath of allegiance to the new government and was accordingly deprived of all his appointments. The enforced freedom from official duties enabled him to carry on his anatomical work with even greater ardour. In 1805 Napoleon passed through Padua on his way to Milan to be crowned King of Italy. Scarpa was not among those who waited to pay homage to the conqueror and Napoleon asked why. Told he would not take the oath, the Emperor exclaimed: "What do political opinions matter in such a case? Scarpa is an honour to the University and to my dominions and I wish him to resume his place". Scarpa was decorated by Napoleon and by the Empress of Austria and honoured by learned societies in many countries. He became F.R.S. in 1791. When the sick Empress of Austria sent for him he was conducted across the Tyrol, then the seat of war, under a flag of truce.

It was in his book, "Ligature of Arteries" (1817), that he described his famous triangle, the femoral or Scarpa's triangle in the thigh, formed by the sartorious and adductor longus muscles and the inguinal (Poupart's) ligament. He also wrote a work on diseases of the eye, which went through five editions, and on club foot and aneurism. He himself regarded his great work on hernia as his masterpiece. He was a talented artist and illustrated many of his own books.

Scarpa was tall and well-built, with sharp features, compressed lips and piercing black eyes. His portrait shows resolution and confidence in every feature. He had a vigorous constitution and was fond of field sports and country life. Reserved and austere in manner, he never married and his life was his work. He accumulated a large fortune from his practice but was no miser and spent his money in forming a collection of works of art. He had a wide knowledge of literature and spoke several languages, but always lectured in Latin. Scarpa died on 31st October 1832 of calculous nephritis. His career shows what can be done with slender clinical resources, properly used, for the observations which made him world-famous were made in a hospital of only 300 beds.

THE SCHICK TEST
Béla Schick 1877-1967

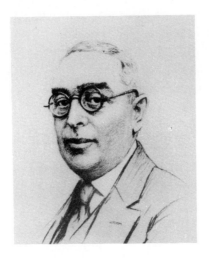

BÉLA SCHICK was born prematurely at Boglar in Hungary on 6th July 1877, when his mother was on a visit to her uncle there, but spent his early years at Graz, Austria. He went to the Staats-Gymnasium in Graz and later to the Karl Franz University where he gained his M.D. in 1900.

At the children's clinic in Graz he worked as an intern with Theodore Escherich and Clemens von Pirquet. When Escherich became director of paediatrics in Vienna he invited von Pirquet and Schick to join him. Schick began his studies on diphtheria in 1906 and in 1913, when privat-dozent in the clinic of von Pirquet, announced his epoch-making discovery of the skin test for diphtheria immunity. He injected into the skin 1/50th of the minimum lethal dose of toxin for a guinea pig. Since 1/30th of a unit of antitoxin per ml of blood is sufficient to neutralise this amount of toxin, a child with less than this amount develops an area of inflammation at the site of the injection. A negative response to the test means the presence of antitoxin in sufficient amount to prevent diphtheria.

Vast numbers of children were Schick-tested in campaigns to eradicate diphtheria and one of Schick's treasures was an album which contained the signatures of one million children who received the Schick test in the New York campaign. That Schick was a great humanitarian and scientist is shown by the award to him of the Addingham gold medal for "the most valuable discovery for relieving pain and suffering humanity".

Schick left Vienna in 1923 to become director of paediatrics at Mount Sinai Hospital, New York, where he remained until his retirement in 1942. He was also director of paediatrics at Sea View Hospital, Staten Island, New York and clinical professor of diseases of children in the postgraduate faculty of Columbia University from 1928-1942. He travelled widely and on one of his visits to South America, at the age of 90, he was stricken with pleurisy on 19th November 1967. He was brought back to New York where he died on 6th December 1967 in Mount Sinai Hospital which he had served so well.

Schick had many delightful attributes which included "the therapy of a smile". Before examining a child he always played with him first. Sometimes he would crouch on the floor and pretend to be a bunny: "You have to be a little childish yourself to be a good paediatrician", he said. His best-known saying was that the physician's best remedy was "tincture of time". He realised how short human memory was and advised every chief of service to have a pet dog which he should leave when retiring from the department which he served: "When you return the only one who will remember you will be your dog".

SIMMONDS'S DISEASE
Morris Simmonds 1855-1925

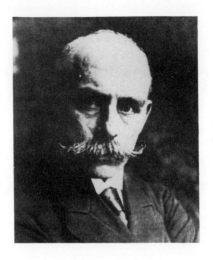

THERE is considerable confusion about what has come to be known as Simmonds's disease. In 1914, in a paper entitled "Ueber Hypophysisschwund mit tödlichem Ausgang" ("Concerning hypophyseal atrophy with fatal outcome"), Deutsche Medizinische Wochenschrift 1914 40 322, Simmonds described the clinical and pathological findings in the case of a married woman of 46 who died in coma after 11 years of ill-health following puerperal sepsis. Menstruation had never returned and she was pale, grey and always weak. All the organs, including the pituitary, were atrophic. Simmonds attributed her condition to septic necrosis of the pituitary. In later papers he suggested the name "pituitary cachexia". This was unfortunate because loss of weight is not an essential feature and its inclusion probably caused some cases of anorexia nervosa to be diagnosed as Simmonds's disease. Although his patient lived 11 years with the disease Simmonds called the condition a "fatal hypophyseal cachexia", but this would be far from accurate today. Indeed, after the pituitary has been completely ablated replacement therapy can nowadays keep the patient free from the effects of pituitary deficiency.

The two common causes of chronic pituitary failure are post-partum necrosis and tumours above the sella turcica, both of which destroy the gland. The post-partum cases are sometimes called Sheehan's syndrome (Sheehan H. L. Quarterly Journal of Medicine 1939 8 277) and the others, Simmonds's disease. This can occur in both sexes. It was in 1939 that the German Medical Society proposed, on the suggestion of Lichtwitz, that anterior pituitary deficiency should be called Simmonds's disease.

Morris Simmonds's forbears came from Denmark and he was born on 14th January 1855 on the then Danish island of St Thomas (now one of the Virgin Islands purchased by the U.S. Government in 1917). Most of the Jews in the Virgin Islands came from Spain and Portugal but none of these were called Simmonds and it is thought that the parents of Morris Simmonds (Colmand Simmonds and Esther, daughter of Moses Abraham Jesurun y Senior) came from Germany. They moved to Hamburg in 1861. Morris left school in 1874 and studied at the universities of Tübingen, Leipzig, Munich and Kiel, passing the state examination at Kiel in 1879. Later he became established as a general practitioner in Hamburg. But his real interest was pathology and he managed to pursue this as well as his practice. He had only modest equipment at the Hospital of St George and not until 1900 did he have a trained assistant. By 1905 his department was properly housed. Post-mortem sessions were held at noon each day and, at the end of each, Simmonds collected all the endocrine organs for study. He showed his talents also in organisation and did much to upgrade the pathology departments of non-teaching hospitals in Germany. He was secretary of the German Pathological Society for many years. In 1909 he gave up his practice and was made "prosektor" (a full-time civil servant). When Hamburg University was opened in 1919 Simmonds was made professor honoris causa.

Simmonds was held in great respect in all the circles in which he moved, not only for his research, but for his personal qualities. In the "Festrede" on his 70th birthday there were expressions of his "ability and generosity". Theodor Rencke, the superintendent of his hospital, described the main traits of Simmonds as "koennen undgoennen", meaning a man who can do well enough himself and never begrudges anybody the credit for what he has done. Simmonds had a happy marriage but his three sons died before him. In spite of this, and the Parkinson's disease which he developed, he was never heard to complain. He walked the six kilometres to St George's Hospital every day. A generous, unselfish and humble man, he died on 25th September 1925.

SJÖGREN'S SYNDROME
Henrik Sjögren born 1889

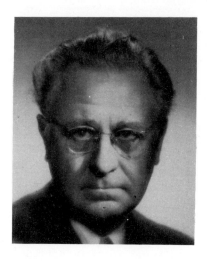

THIS syndrome usually occurs in menopausal women and is a triad consisting of kerato-conjunctivitis sicca (dry eyes), xerostomia (dry mouth) with or without salivary gland enlargement, and, in half to two-thirds of patients, rheumatoid arthritis or some other connective tissue disorder. This "sicca complex" was first described by W. H. Haden in a woman with dry mouth and few tears in his paper, "On dry mouth or suppression of the salivary and buccal secretions" (Transactions of the Clinical Society of London 1888 21 176).

There were other case reports but the first comprehensive account was given by Sjögren (Zur Kenntnis der Kerato-conjunctivitis sicca. Acta Ophthalmologica, Copenhagen 1933 2 1). The term, Sjögren's syndrome, was first used by Bruce Hamilton of Hobart, Tasmania. One of the components of the syndrome, "filamentary conjunctivitis", described by Sjögren is brought out by instilling one per cent Rose Bengal which shows that the filaments consist of mucus and corneal debris. Sjögren also showed that inhalation of ammonia failed to stimulate the secretion of tears. Sometimes the name Mikulicz-Sjögren syndrome, is used but this should be avoided as the conditions described by the two authors are different. Sjögren's syndrome, an auto-immune condition, is occasionally part of the syndrome of Mikulicz (1850-1905) in which there is enlargement of the lachrymal and salivary glands, usually due to sarcoidosis or leukaemia.

Henrik Sjögren was born in the small town of Köping at the western end of Lake Malaren in Sweden on 23rd April 1889. He first attended the local school and then the grammar school at Vasteras. His special interest was music and his favourite instrument the violin. After finishing school in 1918 he began his medical studies at the Caroline Institute in Stockholm. Near the end of his medical course he was invited to be an assistant in the eye clinic and it was then that he saw the first patient with the condition now associated with his name. She was an arthritic complaining of very dry eyes and mouth. After collecting 20 cases of the condition Sjögren wrote his paper. In 1935 he became medical superintendent of the eye clinic at Jönköping. Here he was a pioneer in corneal transplantation and his clinic became a centre for this work. In 1957 Sjögren became lecturer in Professor Rosengren's clinic in Gothenburg and in 1961 the Swedish government conferred on him the title of professor honoris causa.

Professor Sjögren has been invited to visit and give lectures at ophthalmic clinics in many parts of the world. He is now retired and lives in the old university town of Lund.

STILL'S DISEASE
Sir George Frederick Still 1868-1941

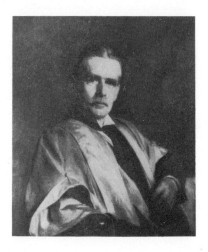

THE title of the thesis which George Frederick Still submitted in 1896 for the degree of M.D. Cambridge was "A special form of joint disease met with in children", the substance of which appeared later in Medico-Chirurgical Transactions 1907 80 47. The thesis was based on a study of 22 cases almost all of which were observed at the Hospital for Sick Children, Great Ormond Street, London, where Still was medical registrar and pathologist. Nineteen of the cases had been under his personal care. This description established the entity of rheumatoid disease in children which has since been known as Still's disease.

Still was born in Holloway, London, on 27th February 1868, the son of George Still, a surveyor for H.M. Customs. He was educated at the Merchant Taylors' School and Gonville and Caius College, Cambridge, where he obtained a First in Classics. His clinical training was at Guy's Hospital. In 1899 he was appointed physician in diseases of children to King's College Hospital — the

first teaching hospital to have a separate paediatric department.
Later he became the first professor of paediatrics in Britain.

When Still started to work with sick children the practice of
paediatrics depended solely on clinical acumen and experience,
but he lived to see the dawn of an era of scientific child care and
became the most celebrated paediatrician of his time. Although he
had a very busy practice he never neglected his hospital work. He
received many honours and in 1937 became physician
extraordinary to H.M. the King and was knighted. Two
appointments which he held gave him vast experience of child
care at the time: those of physician to Dr Barnado's Homes and to
the Society for Waifs and Strays.

Still's best-known writings were "Common Diseases in
Children (5th edition, 1927) and "Common Happenings in
Childhood" (1938). His many-sided personality had a vein of
poetry in it and his "Childhood and Other Poems" (1941) was a
new edition with additions of poems which he had previously
published privately. He was a classical scholar and in 1931 wrote
"Carmen Scholae Medicinae" for the centenary of King's College
Hospital Medical School, and this was set to music and sung at the
celebrations.

Some insight into Still's character can be gained from his poem,
"Life's Aftermath" — the memory of himself he wished to leave
behind.

When I shall die and in the quiet earth
Am laid to rest,
Will there remain some breath of aftermath
Of worst or best,
Some potency of evil or of good,
Its source unguessed
From words or deeds, remembered or forgot,
A life's bequest?
God in his mercy grant that all the wrong
May cease to be,
Not only be forgiven but blotted out,
That so of me
Shall nothing live that might work other's ill,
No legacy
Of harm to lead one single soul astray,
— Thus may it be
When I shall die.

Still is described as being handsome of feature and slight of build, with a grave courtesy all his own. He was no lover of sport but in later life was a rather inefficient dry-fly fishermen, though later he gave this up — probably due to his aversion to taking any form of life. He was unmarried and lived with his widowed mother. He died, aged 73, on 28th June, 1941, at Harnham Croft, Salisbury, Wiltshire.

STOKES—ADAMS ATTACKS
CHEYNE—STOKES BREATHING
William Stokes 1804-1878

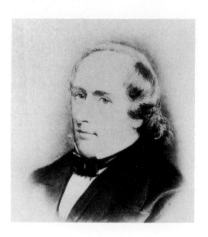

WILLIAM STOKES's name has become eponymous on two counts, in neither of which did he make the original observation. But his writings brought both of them to the notice of the medical world when they might otherwise have been forgotten. In his paper, "Observations on Some Cases of Permanently Slow Pulse" (Dublin Quarterly Journal of Medical Science 1846 2 73-85), he dealt entirely with this clinical disorder. He referred to a paper of Adams 19 years earlier on "Cases of Diseases of the Heart accompanied with Pathological Observations" (Dublin Hospital Reports 1827 4 353) in which one case of slow pulse was mentioned among many other conditions. As credit generally goes to the man who convinces the world of his work, the eponym Stokes—Adams attacks seems fairer than Adams—Stokes attacks if fullness, and not merely priority, of description is the criterion. Priority alone would award the eponym to Marcus Gerbezius who described syncope in temporary cardiac arrest in 1691 (Pulsus mira inconstantia. Misc. cur. Ephem. nat. cur. Norimbergae 1692 10 115-118) or to Morgagni who described it in 'de Sedibus" in 1781.

In 1854 Stokes extended the description of rhythmic breathing originally described by John Cheyne in 1818 and now referred to as Cheyne—Stokes respiration. It occurs in two groups of patients — those with intra-cranial disease and those with cardiac disease. It is thought that two main factors cause it — prolongation of the circulation time and altered sensitivity of the respiratory centre, but the exact mechanism is still somewhat obscure.

William Stokes's father, Whitley Stokes, was regius professor of medicine at Dublin University and physician to the Meath Hospital. He was especially fond of his son, William, and they used to go on scientific and archeological expeditions in the Irish hills. These excursions into natural history developed William's powers of observation. He studied clinical medicine with his father at the Meath Hospital before becoming a student in Edinburgh where he graduated M.D. in 1825, and in the same year he published a small treatise on the stethoscope. He returned to Dublin to be physician to the Dublin General Dispensary and was later elected to the staff of the Meath Hospital in succession to his father. Here he reorganised the teaching and insisted that an arts degree was necessary before admission as a medical student, saying: "Let us emancipate the student and give him time and opportunity for the cultivation of his mind". Stokes was a lover of art and had many distinguished visitors to his home in Dublin. He began his day's work at 4 or 5 a.m., and said: "My father left me but one legacy, the blessed gift of rising early".

WHIPPLE'S DISEASE
George Hoyt Whipple 1878-1976

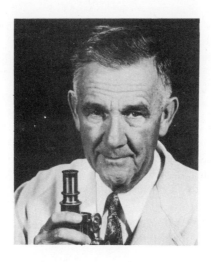

THE work which gave Whipple's disease its eponymous name was done very early in Whipple's career when he was an instructor in pathology at Johns Hopkins University. His first research was largely histological and included a rare case of what he described as intestinal lipodystrophy. The patient was a 37-year-old medical missionary who had suffered for over five years in Turkey from loss of weight, fatty stools, vague abdominal symptoms and multiple arthritis. On return to the U.S.A. in 1907 he was admitted to the Johns Hopkins Hospital as a possible case of Hodgkin's disease and died after laparotomy. Whipple reported the case as a "a hitherto undescribed disease in the intestinal and mesenteric lymphatic tissues" (Bulletin of the Johns Hopkins Hospital 1907 18 382). Clinically it is characterised by diarrhoea, steatorrhoea and lymphadenopathy. Jejunal biopsy (not possible in 1905) shows macrophages laden with what is now known to be glycoprotein. Recent work suggests that it may be caused by bacterial infection and some cases have responded to antibiotics. It is a rare disorder, only about 200 cases having been described, but more than that number of papers have been written about it.

George Hoyt Whipple* was born on 28th August 1878 at Ashland in the lake district of New Hampshire. His father and grandfather were general practitioners. He grew up in the country and always remained interested in rural pursuits. His father died when he was two years old and his mother and grandmother Hoyt took great interest in his education. This was at schools in Ashland and later in nearby Tilton and finally at the Academy in Andover.

He obtained his A.B. in 1900 at Yale where he found biochemistry exciting. Without being influenced in any way he always said he would be a doctor. He was keen on athletics and, before starting his medical studies, he spent a year at a military academy at Ossining, New York, where he taught science and was in charge of athletics. His main purpose, however, was to earn money to make himself self-supporting during his student years. He began his medical studies at Johns Hopkins University in 1901 and spent the summer vacations working on the steamers on the lakes of New Hampshire.

With the exception of one year, 1907-08, as pathologist to the Ancon Hospital in Panama, where he came into contact with General Gorgas, Dr Whipple was at the Johns Hopkins Medical School from 1905 to 1914, becoming associate professor. He married in 1914 and moved to San Francisco where he was professor of research medicine at the University of California Medical School in the year 1920-21. After this he became professor of pathology and dean of the School of Medicine and Dentistry at the University of Rochester when the new medical school was started. Here he began to study the influence of food on blood regeneration in dogs rendered anaemic by bleeding. He found that some foods stimulated the marrow more than others and especially liver. This established liver therapy for pernicious

---

*Whipple's triad of symptoms in hypoglycaemia is named after A. O. Whipple a friend of W. H. Whipple.

anaemia and subsequently led to the isolation of vitamin B^{12}. Whipple was president of the American Association of Pathology and Bacteriology in 1930 and received many awards and honours including the Nobel Prize in 1934 which he shared with George Minot and William Murphy. In 1932 he had investigated Mediterranean anaemia and proposed the term thalassaemia. Research and teaching were the cornerstones of Whipple's career, bringing him satisfaction and happiness. It is as a teacher that he wished to be remembered.

KINNIER WILSON'S DISEASE
WILSON'S SIGN
S. A. Kinnier Wilson 1878-1937

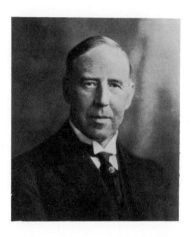

SAMUEL ALEXANDER KINNIER WILSON, the only son of the Rev.
James Kinnier Wilson, of Co. Monaghan, Ireland, was born on
6th December 1878 at Cedarville, New Jersey, U.S.A. The family
soon moved to Scotland. "Sam" was educated at George Watson's
College and Edinburgh University, obtaining the degrees of M.A.
(1897), M.B. (1902) and B.Sc. in physiology with first-class
honours (1903). He was Carnegie Fellow in Paris for a year and
studied under Pierre Marie and Babinski at the Pitié. Then, after a
brief visit to Leipzig, he went to The National Hospital for the
Relief and Cure of the Paralysed and Epileptic, London* where he
occupied various posts for a total of 33 years. He was one of a
group of famous neurologists which included Gowers and
Hughlings Jackson.

---

*The name was changed in 1926 to The National Hospital, Queen Square, for the
Relief and Cure of Diseases of the Nervous System including Paralysis and
Epilepsy and again, in 1948, to The National Hospital for Nervous Diseases.

Tetanoid chorea associated with cirrhosis of the liver had been mentioned by W. R. Gowers in his manual of Diseases of the Nervous System in 1888 but it was Wilson's famous monograph, entitled "Progressive Lenticular Degeneration: a Familial Disease associated with Cirrhosis of the Liver", published in Brain (1912 34 295), which brought clinical and pathological recognition of this condition.

Wilson was still a registrar at the time and his paper gained him the degree of M.D. with gold medal and also an international reputation. It was the first study of disease in the extrapyramidal system and was based on four examples personally observed, with notes on the unpublished cases of others. Wilson's work was better known abroad than that of other British neurologists, for he was fluent in French and German and a man of Olympian stature in the neurological world between World Wars I and II. His lectures had always a dramatic and compelling quality and did much to enhance the great reputation of "Queen Square" as a teaching centre. One of his mannerisms was to roll up the collar of his white coat and bring the lapels together under his chin and then fold his arms across his chest before proceeding with his lecture.

Wilson's contributions to neurology were many in addition to the description of the disease which bears his name. His Croonian lectures in 1925 on "Disorders of Motility and Muscle Tone" and his Harveian Oration in 1926 on "The Epilepsies" have the qualities of greatness. In 1920 he founded the Journal of Neurology and Psychopathology and he was president of the Section of Neurology of the Royal Society of Medicine from 1933 to 1935. He died on 12th May 1937 — unfortunately, before he had quite completed his massive textbook of neurology. After his death the work was finished and edited by A. Ninian Bruce and chapter 47 of volume 2 is on "Hepato-lenticular Degeneration". The disease is now known to be a rare recessively inherited condition in which an error of copper metabolism leads to the deposition of the metal in the brain and liver.

Wilson's name has been given also to the sign of the positive glabellar tap in early Parkinsonism. Tapping the root of the nose causes blinking which persists with each tap, whereas it normally ceases after a few taps. (Reflex blinking from visual threat is avoided by making the tapping finger invisible).

FOR FURTHER READING

ADAMS   Obituary. *Lancet* (1875). *1* 145.
ADDISON   Ober, W. B. (1973). *Great Men of Guy's.*
                 History of Medicine series No. 42. Metuchen
                 Scarecrow Reprint Corp.
ADIE   Obituary. *British Medical Journal* (1935). *2*
                 629.
BABINSKI   Miller, H. (1967). *Three Great Neurologists.*
                 Proceedings of the Royal Society of Medicine.
                 60 399.
BELL   Gordon-Taylor, G. and Walls, H. W. (1958).
                 Sir Charles Bell, his life and times. Edinburgh.
                 Livingstone.
BOWMAN   Hale-White, W. (1935). *Great Doctors of the*
                 Nineteenth Century. London. Edward
                 Arnold.
BROCA   Gibson, W. G. (1962). *Pioneers in localisation*
                 of function in the Brain. Journal of the
                 American Medical Association. 180 944.
BRUCE   James, T. (1970). *Sir David Bruce Bt, F.R.S. A*
                 Memoir. South African Medical Journal. 44
                 1098.
BUERGER   *Who's Who Among Physicians and Surgeons*
                 New York (1938). *1* 157.
BURKITT   Bernard Glemser (1971). *The Long Safari.*
                 London. The Bodley Head.
CALMETTE   *Obituary Notices of the Royal Society* (1934). *3*
                 315.
CASTELLANI   Aldo Castellani (1960). *Microbes, Men and*
                 Monarchs. London. Gollancz.
CHARCOT   Tomlinson, J. C. and Haymaker, W. (1957).
                 Archives of Neurology. 77 44.
CHEYNE   Willius, F. A. and Keys, T. E. (1941). *Cardiac*
                 Classics. London. Kimpton.
CONN   Conn, Jerome W. (1961). *Blood, Sweat, Tears*
                 — and other Biological Fluids. Michigan
                 Alumnus Quarterly Review. 67 21.

CROHN   *Medicine's Living History. Medical World News.* (1972). 2 Aug. page 33.

CUSHING   Fulton, J. F. (1946). *Harvey Cushing, a biography.* Springfield. Chas. C. Thomas.

DARWIN   Dobson, Jessie (1959). *Charles Darwin and Down House.* Edinburgh. Livingstone.

DOWN   Payne, R. (1965). *The Centenary of Mongolism. Journal of Mental Subnormality.* 2 89.

DUPUYTREN   Haeston, J. T. (1960). Baron Dupuytren. *The Medical Journal of Australia.* 1 808.

FALLOT   Willius, F. A. and Keys, T. E. (1941). *Cardiac Classics.* London. Kimpton.

GUÉRIN   *Revue de Tuberculose et de Pneumologie* (1961). 25 695.

HANSEN   Feeny, P. (1964). *The Fight against Leprosy.* London. Elek Books.

HARVEY   Kcele, K. D. (1965). *William Harvey, The Man, The Physician and The Scientist.* London. Nelson.

HASHIMOTO   Doniach, D. and Roitt, I. M. (1962). *The Lancet.* 1 1074.

HODGKIN   Morrison, H. (1956). *Doctors Afield: Thomas Hodgkin. Guy's Hospital Gazette.* 70 358.

HORNER   Wood, Casey A. ed (1916). *American Encyclopaedia and Dictionary of Ophthalmology. vol. 3.* Chicago. Cleveland Press.

HUNTINGTON   de Jong, R. N. (1937). *Annals of Medical History.* 201.

JACKSON   Hutchinson, J. (1911). *Recollections of a Lifelong Friendship. British Medical Journal* 2 1551.

KOPLIK   Bass, M.H. (1955). *Pediatric Profiles. Henry Koplik. Journal of Pediatrics.* 46 119.

KORSAKOV   Victor, M. and Yakovlev, P.I. (1955). *S. S. Korsakov's Psychic Disorder in Conjunction with Peripheral Neuritis. Neurology (Minneapolis).* 5 394.

McARDLE   Holling, H. E. (1965). *The Birth of a Syndrome. Annals of Internal Medicine. 62* 412.

MACEWEN   Bowman, A. K. (1942). *The Life and Teaching of Sir William Bowman.* Glasgow. Hodge.

MANSON   Manson-Bahr, P. and Alcock, A. (1927). *The Life and Work of Sir Patrick Manson.* London Cassell.

MECKEL   Meader, R. G. (1937). *The Meckel Dynasty in Medical Education. Yale Journal of Biology and Medicine. 10* 1.

MENIÈRE   Stothers, H. H. (1961). *Prosper Menière, The Centenary of an Eponym. Annals of Otology* (St. Louis). *70* 319.

de MORGAN   Plarr, V. G. (1930). *Lives of Fellows of the Royal College of Surgeons of England. 1* 331.

OSLER   Cushing, Harvey (1925). *The Life of Sir William Osler.* 2 volumes Oxford. Clarendon Press.

PAGET   Bett, W. R. (1925). *The Life and Works of Sir James Paget. St. Bartholomew's Hospital Journal. 33* 21.

PARKINSON   McMenemy, W. H. (1935). *James Parkinson Centenary Volume.* London. Macmillan.

PAUL   Bett, W. R. (1951). *Frank Thomas Paul. Annals of the Royal College of Surgeons. 9* 408.

POTT   Dobson, Jessie (1972). *Annals of the Royal College of Surgeons. 50* 1.

RAMSTEDT   Obituary. *The Lancet* (1963). *1* 674.

RAYNAUD   *Journal of The American Medical Association. Maurice Raynaud (1834-1881) Raynaud's Disease.* (1967). *200* 985.

REITER   Owen, D. S. Jnr., (1972). *Reiter and his Syndrome. Virginia Medical Monthly. 99* 267.

ROBERTSON   Obituary. *British Medical Journal* (1909). *1* 191.

ROMBERG   Burr, R. W. (1942). *New England Journal of Medicine. 227* 566.

RYLE   Obituary. *British Medical Journal* (1950). *1* 611.

SCARPA   Morris, M. (1896). *The Practitioner. Heroes of Medicine series.* 57 168.

SCHICK   Kagan, S. R. (1945). *The Modern Medical World.* Boston.

SIMMONDS   Griesbach, W. E. (1965). *Morris Simmonds, Pioneer Endocrinologist — Some Recollections. Journal of Endocrinology.* 25 1671.

SJÖGREN   Sjögren, H. and Bloch, K. J. (1971). *Survey of Ophthalmology* 16 No. 3 145.

STILL   Thursfield, H. (1941). *In Memoriam: George Frederick Still. Archives of Disease in Childhood. 16* 147.

STOKES   Willius, F. A. and Keys, T. E. (1941) *Cardiac Classics.* London. Kimpton.

WHIPPLE   Whipple, G. H. (1959). *Autobiographical Sketch. Perspectives in Biology Vol 2* (Spring).

WILSON   Haymaker, W. and Schiller, F. (1970). *Founders of Neurology. 2nd edition.* Springfield. Chas. C. Thomas.

INDEX

Names and page numbers in bold type indicate the main biography

Names We Remember

Names We Remember